A
Natural
Mistake

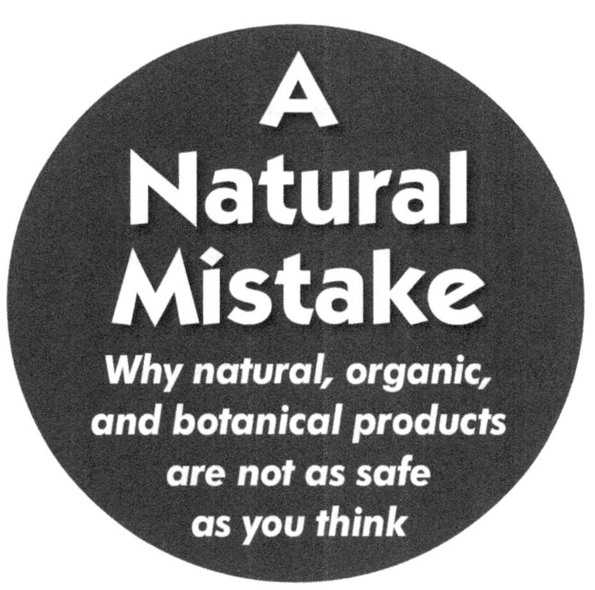

James T. MacGregor, Ph.D., D.A.B.T.

A Natural Mistake

Copyright © 2019 James T. MacGregor

Disclaimer
Despite the author's considerable experience in product
regulation and safety evaluation and best efforts to assure
accuracy, the absence of factual errors cannot be guaranteed.
It is important to recognize that scientific and regulatory
information are not static, but constantly change as new
scientific information becomes available and regulations
are updated or modified. Readers should not base decisions
concerning product choices, health practices, or regulatory
modifications solely on the information presented herein,
but should also consider information from
other authoritative sources.

ISBN# Softcover: 978-1-7333880-0-9
E-book: 978-1-7333880-1-6

Cover design by Deborah Perdue,
Illumination Graphics, www.illuminationgraphics.com

Cover photos courtesy of www.depositphotos.com
and www.shutterstock.com

About the Cover

The cover shows some of the many natural products that have caused health problems. From top to bottom:

Grapefruit contains a potent inhibitor of the enzyme responsible for breaking down a number of important drugs, which can cause toxicity at normally safe doses due to increased blood levels

St. John's wort, commonly used as a botanical supplement for its antidepressant properties, accelerates the metabolic breakdown of certain drugs and has caused the rejection of surgical transplants by inactivating the drug used to prevent immune rejection

Fava beans are widely consumed as food but are toxic to individuals who have a specific mutant gene

Botanical supplements, represented by the capsules, are particularly dangerous because they can be sold with little or no safety testing and are frequently adulterated with biologically active chemicals

Açaí berries are widely sought for their antioxidant properties, even though they contain far higher levels of the same type of chemicals used as preservatives that many seek to avoid

About the Author

The author's career has been devoted to the development, safety evaluation, and regulation of pharmaceutical and food products. He is a Diplomate of the American Board of Toxicology and has been President of the Regulatory and Safety Evaluation Specialty Section of the Society of Toxicology, President of the Association of Government Toxicologists, and president of other national and regional professional societies involved with product safety testing. He has been Director of the Office of Testing and Research at the Food and Drug Administration's Center for Drug Evaluation and Research and Director of the Washington Office of the National Center for Toxicological Research, Rockville, MD, Director of the Toxicology and Metabolism Laboratory of SRI International (formerly the Stanford Research Institute), in Menlo Park, CA, and Director of Food Safety Research at the U.S. Department of Agriculture Western Regional Research Center, Albany, CA. He was an Adjunct Associate Professor in the School of Public Health at the University of California, Berkeley, an Adjunct Faculty member at the University of San Francisco, and has been a guest lecturer in toxicology training programs at these universities and at the University of California School of Medicine, San Francisco, and the U.S. Food and Drug Administration, Rockville and College Park, MD. He holds a Ph.D. in Toxicology from the University of Rochester School of Medicine and Dentistry, a Bachelor of Science in Chemistry from Union College, and completed post-doctoral training at the University of California School of Medicine, San Francisco. He has published more than 200 articles and chapters in scientific journals and books, has served on numerous national and international professional committees in the field of product safety, and has been a frequent invited speaker at national and international scientific meetings.

Table of Contents

Chapter 1
Introduction

Several years ago, while working at the Food and Drug Administration (FDA) in the Center responsible for drug product review and research, I became involved in a situation that came to be an important motivation for undertaking this book. Because of my experience as a toxicologist, the Center responsible for the safety of foods and botanical products invited me to participate in a committee that reviewed reports to the FDA of potential adverse effects associated with the use of botanical supplements. One of the early reports considered by this committee was a case in which a young healthy teenage girl with an outstanding academic record died abruptly and unexpectedly after beginning to take a botanical product. The FDA official presenting this case indicated that the case had been discussed with FDA legal staff, and the conclusion was that there would not be a basis for any legal action without additional evidence that the death was in fact caused by the botanical agent. The attorneys, of course, were correct in concluding that a single case in which an exposure and effect appear to be associated, even the abrupt death of a young healthy teenager, is only circumstantial evidence that the exposure was in fact the cause of the death. Some other unknown factor may have been responsible.

This legal opinion was not surprising to me, but the ensuing follow-up to this case dramatically illustrated the sharp contrast between the rigorous requirements for safety, identity, and impurity content required by the Center where I was working for approval to sell pharmaceutical products and the minimal requirements that applied to botanical products. The committee and the responsible FDA division did follow up by looking to see if other reports of toxicity with similar or related products had been received, and the FDA conducted chemical analyses of products believed to be similar or identical to the responsible product and performed some minimal toxicity studies of those products at their laboratories. However, conclusions were hampered by the lack of knowledge of the exact composition of the product in question due to the absence of rigorous standards for chemical identity, composition, purity, and method of production. The FDA did not have a sample of the actual product taken by the teenager and did not have the resources to conduct extensive safety evaluation studies of the type that would have been required of a food additive, pesticide, or pharmaceutical agent. Nor did they believe that they could compel the manufacturer or business that sold the supplement to conduct the necessary studies. At least during the period of my involvement with this case, the FDA was unable either to reach a conclusion about whether the product in question was causally associated with this young girl's death or to follow up with studies designed to determine if the product in question was a serious health risk.

As I learned more about the shortcomings of the safety laws that applied to botanical products, and witnessed more cases of potential adverse reactions to dietary supplements reported to the FDA, I became increasingly aware of the need for a book such as this to make the public more aware of the health risks associated with dietary supplement products.

Sales of dietary supplements have grown dramatically. In 2019 the FDA estimated that 50,000 to 80,000 different dietary supplement products were on the market (U.S. Food and Drug Administration, 2019). This is an extraordinary growth from the approximately 4000 products estimated to be on the market in 1994, the year that the Dietary Supplement Health and Education Act (DSHEA) was enacted. This Act, which made it possible to market such products with minimal safety evaluation, will be discussed in more detail in subsequent chapters.   In monetary terms, a recent survey showed that the annual sales of herbal dietary supplements in the U.S. have grown to more than seven billion dollars, not counting sales of government-approved herbal drug products, botanical ingredients in cosmetics, and most herbal teas. Of these sales, 17% were through mass market outlets such as supermarkets, drug stores, and military commissaries, 34% through natural and health food stores, and 48% through direct sales to consumers such as *via* the internet, direct mail, and direct response to radio and TV ads. In addition to real and serious health risks from herbal supplements, the burgeoning market for "natural" and "organic" foods is costing consumers inflated prices for products touted as more healthful and safe when in fact careful scientific review of the evidence does not substantiate the health and safety claims. Market basket surveys by consumer groups and government agencies substantiate what every shopper already knows–that organic foods are more expensive than "conventional" foods.   For example, a survey of 100 different product types by Consumer Reports in 2015 found that organic products were on average 47% more expensive than conventional products, but that the range was large with the organic products sometimes costing twice or more as much (Consumer Reports, 2015). Correspondingly, the U.S.

Department of Agriculture Economic Research Service has surveyed wholesale prices of fruits and vegetables and found organic products to be generally in the range of 20-180% more expensive than conventional products (USDA, Updated 2016).

There is widespread belief that natural supplements and herbal remedies are safer and more beneficial than drug products made by large pharmaceutical companies and that organic foods are more healthful than those produced using pesticides, artificial preservatives, and manufactured fertilizers. This belief is based largely on the supposition that products made by nature are inherently safe and beneficial and that synthetic chemicals made by man are generally toxic and should be avoided. Contrary to these widely held views, the current regulations that apply to food additives, pesticides, and pharmaceuticals require extensive safety testing and regulatory review, as well as very conservative assumptions that establish safe levels allowed in final products. In contrast, natural botanical dietary supplements, nutraceutical products, and new food crop varieties bred to elevate naturally occurring biologically active chemical constituents for pest and disease resistance can generally be sold with minimal or sometimes no specific safety testing. Further, botanical supplements are frequently adulterated with illegal biologically active chemicals or drugs and the prevailing law controlling dietary supplements places the major responsibility for identifying and controlling dangerous products on the Food and Drug Administration without providing the resources and funding necessary to implement effective controls.

Many cases of severe toxicity and deaths from natural products have been documented, but widespread misunderstanding of the relative safety of natural products persists. In fact, natural products generally have a far lower level of safety assurance than do the conventional products about which most consumers seem to worry. Given the many cases of severe toxicity that have occurred from natural botanical products, and extensive evidence that they are frequently adulterated with dangerous bioactive substances, one might ask why the belief in the inherent healthfulness of natural products is so strong. This mistaken belief appears to be due largely to reliance on one or more of the following erroneous assumptions:

1. *It is obvious that natural foods are healthful and safe because our very survival and well-being depend on them.*

    Food is essential to our survival and well-being and is therefore generally considered inherently wholesome and ben-eficial—by the public, legislators, and regulatory scientists alike. The fact that food is an integral part of the social fabric of society (serving and enjoying food together is a universal component of hospitality) undoubtedly adds to this perception. Nevertheless even the chemicals and food constituents in the foods essential to our well-being can be toxic at excessively high exposures. It is the combination of each chemical's biological potency and the extent of our exposure to it that determines whether it is safe, beneficial, or harmful. Oxygen, salt, water, and dietary fat are all essential to life but can kill us at exaggerated exposures. It would be an unwise decision indeed to conclude that we should avoid exposure to oxygen, water, and salt because experiments have demonstrated that they can be toxic at excessively high exposures. Conversely, even highly toxic chemicals are safe if the exposure to them is sufficiently low.

2. *Herbal remedies are safer than prescription drugs because they have been used for hundreds of years without reports of signif-icant toxicities, while synthetic pharmaceuticals are known to have many toxic side effects.*

    Although acute toxicities that occur soon after exposure to an agent are easily identified, it is often very difficult to associate adverse effects that are delayed or that depend on interaction with another agent or physiological condition. Because the law governing the safety of natural botanical supplements allows them to be sold without the requirement that they be tested for these latter types of toxicity, it is generally unknown whether these types of toxicity occur. Unlike botanical supplements, pharmaceuticals must be thoroughly tested for all types of toxicity before they can be sold, and this includes testing at higher and higher doses until toxicity is achieved or no more can be given. This is done so that the exposure levels at which potential toxicities occur can be known and therefore lower allowable exposures can be established so that any potential toxicities do not occur during normal use. This requirement for testing at exaggerated doses to assure that adequate safety margins can be set means that there are almost always reports of toxicities of drug products. In the case of botanical products there are far fewer reports of toxicity because this high-exposure testing has not been done and many potential toxicities therefore remain unknown. Thus, critical safety margins that assure a lack of toxicity have not been established. There are numerous examples of serious and fatal effects of botanical products that have occurred in humans, and laboratory studies have shown that many natural chemical constituents of plants or herbal products are toxic.

3. *Synthetic pesticides are toxic by design, so residues in food products must be harmful.*

Although many synthetic pesticides are toxic, their potential toxicities are studied carefully and allowable levels of residues that do not cause toxicity are established using very conservative safety margins. Plants, including food plants, have evolved to produce their own natural pesticides but the requirements for studying and testing these natural pesticides are much less rigorous than those designed and added by man.

Indeed, many currently used commercial pesticides are derived from naturally occurring pesticidal chemicals.

4. *Organic products are more healthful than conventional ones because they are free of toxic pesticide residues and harmful chemical additives.*

    There is no substantial evidence that suggests that organic products are safer or more healthful than conventional products. Allowable levels of additives and pesticide residues are determined by extensive safety testing and substantial safety margins are used to assure that the toxicities observed at exaggerated doses do not occur during normal product use. Organic food products are selected or bred for pest resistance, which is generally associated with higher levels of naturally occurring defensive chemicals in plants, but these resistant varieties do not require special toxicity testing unless there is an *a priori* reason to suspect the presence of toxic constituents.

5. *Genetically modified (GM) or bioengineered (BE) foods or food crops are no longer natural, so products produced by conventional breeding and variety selection are clearly preferred.*

    The focus of FDA and USDA regulations that apply to bioengineered food sources are limited mainly to modern biochemical methods of genetic alteration such as recombinant DNA technology and these regulations specifically exclude genetic modifications introduced by conventional methods of breeding and selection of desired genetic variants. However, conventional breeding and variant selection also introduce genetic alterations and in fact are far less specific than the modern methods of biochemical DNA manipulation. These modern methods can introduce very specific desired changes without the high background of unknown genetic changes associated with the traditional methods, and in addition are more thoroughly tested for possible safety issues than the latter.

6. *All-natural products are preferred because of their greater safety and superior nutritional properties.*

Given the major focus on natural foods, it is perhaps surprising that the FDA has not provided a formal rule or guidance that defines the terms "natural" and "all-natural" or whether these terms have any meaning in terms of health or safety. They have issued a statement that their working definition is that "natural" means nothing artificial or synthetic has been added that wouldn't normally be expected in that food, but have noted that there is not a formal rule or guidance that clarifies whether various changes due to processing, content of genetically modified constituents, use of pesticides, animal husbandry practices, etc., affect whether the term natural should be used in product labeling. The FDA has asked for public input on these issues but has yet to issue a more comprehensive definition. Studies have failed to show any health or safety benefit of organic or natural *vs.* conventional products.

Each of the above assumptions and the reasons that they are erroneous will be discussed in depth in subsequent chapters, including examples of severe toxicities and deaths that have been caused by natural botanical products and the difficulty of identifying the causative agents and of controlling their availability in the marketplace.

Throughout my career, which has been focused on the evaluation and regulation of the safety of food and drug products, I have been aware of the dichotomy between these general beliefs and the wide disparity in actual objective safety studies and regulatory enforcement capabilities that underpin the degree of safety assurance among product classes. The objective of this book is to make available the facts needed by consumers to make better choices among food, drug, and supplement products. Additionally, I am hopeful that legislators and regulatory officials may be motivated by the following discussion to address the need for an improved regulatory approach that enhances consumer safety and provides a more uniform approach to risk assessment and regulation across product classes, as previous writings such as Upton Sinclair's *The Jungle* and Rachel Carson's *Silent Spring* have done.

In my first professional position, initially as a research scientist and then as supervisor of the major food safety research group at the U.S. Department of Agriculture, I learned that all plants, including our major food crops, synthesize thousands of unique biologically active chemicals in order to protect themselves from insect and animal predators and microbial diseases, to inhibit the growth of other plants that compete for nutrients, water, and sunlight, to attract beneficial insects and animals, and to communicate with each other. Many of these are potentially toxic and only the intelligence of the human species and millennia of evolutionary adaptation have made us able to select potentially useful food plants, to breed out undesirable characteristics while retaining food value, and to metabolically detoxify potentially harmful chemical constituents in native plants. In this position we studied many plant constituents with the potential to induce general toxicity as well as the influence of dietary constituents on delayed diseases such as cancer and reproductive defects. The number of plant constituents with the potential to cause such effects led us to place a sign in our laboratory designed to deliver an important message to visitors. It read "Try Aflatoxin, it's Natural". Aflatoxin is a natural toxin so potent that feeding just a few micrograms, or about one ten-millionth of an ounce, per day to rats in laboratory studies is sufficient to cause cancer in virtually all of the exposed animals. The sign could equally well have read "Try hemlock", or "ricin", or "digitalis", or "curare", or "nicotine", or many other highly toxic plants or plant constituents. The natural resistance of plants to predators and diseases is known to be due to many biologically active chemicals that can cause toxicity. However, new cultivars of crop plants bred for increased disease or pest resistance do not require the type of special safety assessments that would be required of a new food additive or pesticide residue unless the plant is already known to have a toxic potential or unless specific genetic manipulation introduces DNA not naturally present in those plant varieties.

In subsequent positions as Director of the SRI International Toxicology Laboratory (the former Stanford Research Institute in Menlo Park, California) and in supervisory positions at the Food and Drug Administration, I had the opportunity to oversee many of the safety studies required to evaluate potential toxicities and to establish safe limits in food and drug products offered for sale. I also served on FDA, national, and international committees involved with product safety evaluation standards and the methodology used to identify adverse health effects. During this period, I came to appreciate the major differences in requirements for safety testing among different classes of products. The regulations governing safety assurance require some products to undergo extensive safety testing and review by the responsible regulatory agency prior to being offered for sale or used as a product constituent, while others are permitted to be sold with little or no safety testing. Further, the burden of proof to establish safety or risk varies widely among different product classes and even among different products within the same class depending on when they were (or are) introduced for sale. In some cases, the burden is on the company manufacturing or selling the product to conduct detailed studies that test for many different types of acute and delayed adverse health effects, including cancer, delayed neurotoxicity, and reproductive effects, and to submit the results for review and approval by the appropriate government agency prior to any sales. In other cases, the product may be sold without government review and the burden is on the government to establish harm or undue risk of harm before it can take regulatory action against an unsafe product.

Unfortunately, the law governing the safety of natural botanical supplements, the Dietary Supplement Health and Education Act of 1994 (DSHEA), allows these products to be sold with little or no safety testing. It also removes from the companies that manufacture or sell these products the burden of proving product safety before they are sold. Instead, the FDA must prove harm or undue risk of harm before regulatory action can be taken against unsafe or adulterated products. The rules and regulations that apply to different products are so complex that even career regulatory scientists generally do not know the details of requirements for products other than those for which they are immediately responsible. It is not surprising that the average consumer often does not have sufficient knowledge to make informed judgments about the relative risks and benefits of different products.

The existing laws and regulatory structure have resulted in a heavy bias in resource allocation toward those products and product constituents that require the demonstration of safety with subsequent regulatory review prior to their sale, rather than dietary supplements that are permitted to be marketed with minimal safety testing and lax identity, purity, and manufacturing standards. The products generally perceived by the public to be of the highest health risk, including food additives, pesticide residues, pharmaceutical products, and medical devices, are in fact those with the most rigorous safety assurance requirements, while natural botanical supplements and natural constituents of food products, which many perceive as inherently safer, receive much less rigorous safety testing. In the case of dietary supplements, the enforcement ability of the FDA is also much more restricted and it is difficult to either mandate or commit internal resources to perform the highly expensive and time-consuming studies necessary to perform a complete safety evaluation of even a single specific product for which there is a potential association with a documented fatality. If a finding similar to the above case occurred with a product class that required the Sponsor to assure safety prior to selling it, then the FDA could request such studies and the responsible company would generally comply. Thus, the difference in the level of safety assurance between natural products and synthetic food additives, pesticide residues, and prescription pharmaceutical products is actually the opposite of that generally perceived by the public.

The balance of resources within the regulatory agency may at first seem counter-intuitive, because one might think that the FDA would prioritize the commitment of resources to the study of those products that are being marketed with the least safety data and not those for which a Sponsor has been required to produce extensive data prior to sale. However on second thought one realizes that not only is the burden on the FDA in each case very different, but that the incentives to the Agency to allocate resources favors a focus on those products for which specific Sponsor studies and FDA review are required prior to the sale of the product. In the case of pharmaceuticals, food additives, and pesticides, the burden is on the Sponsor to demonstrate safety, and the regulatory agency is required to review the results of all the required studies in a timely manner, to prepare formal evaluation reports, and to hold necessary meetings with Sponsors and expert advisory boards. These responsibilities are required, and the Agency is subject to complaints and pressures if they do not execute them in a timely fashion. In the case of less rigorously regulated products, there is no specific mandate that requires that the FDA pursue a specific issue and the resources available for such follow-up studies are much more severely restricted.

Consumers not familiar with how product safety is evaluated and how this process determines the level of safety assurance deserve to know the facts about these issues so they can make informed decisions about the relative benefits and risks associated with different types of products. In subsequent chapters we will look more deeply into the basis and consequences of the "natural mistake" of assuming that natural products are inherently more safe than synthetic ones, including 1) the reasons consumers and legislators have considered natural plant sources of food and dietary supplements to be more safe and wholesome than foods produced with pesticides, food additives, and artificial fertilizers; 2) the reality of scientific knowledge showing that plants naturally synthesize thousands of potentially toxic chemicals with which they combat predators, competitors, and diseases and attract beneficial species needed for pollination and seed dispersal; 3) disparities under current laws and regulations that often provide a higher level of safety assurance for synthetic *vs.* natural chemical constituents—the opposite of that generally believed to be the case; 4) the importance of whether the "burden of proof" of either safety or potential for harm lies with the product manufacturer or vendor or with the responsible regulatory agency, whether prospective safety testing is required prior to selling the product, and whether regulatory action depends on the demonstration that harm has occurred or is likely to occur; and 5) why a history of product use without known toxicities is not adequate evidence of product safety and why only prospective safety testing before marketing can detect certain types of toxicities. The particularly serious problems with dangerous and adulterated botanical supplements and the reasons the 1994 Dietary Supplement Health and Education Act makes adequate regulatory oversight of these products extremely difficult will be given particular emphasis. Examples will be provided that illustrate how serious hazards have often not been identified and why prospective safety evaluation of all classes of ingested products is essential if safety is to be assured.

It is hoped that the reader will take the time to better understand the information presented in subsequent chapters, in order to be able to make better product choices. Equally important, it is hoped that those responsible for product safety legislation and regulatory implementation will take note of the issues raised and become motivated to consider regulatory changes that provide more uniform safety analysis and regulation across different product classes.

Chapter 2
Plants Are Not Benign:
Chemical Warfare and Plant Evolution

Plants are not chemical free. Nor are they benign. Plants contain more than 100,000 chemicals not present in animals, most of which are biologically active and many of which are toxic. These chemicals possess the biological activities necessary for defense of the plant against insect and animal predators, prevention of plant diseases, responses to injury, attraction of favorable species that are beneficial to the plant (such as pollinators or secondary predators that prey on insects that attack the plant), and deterrence of competitive plant species that would otherwise crowd out the plant or deprive it of needed nutrients. Because these specialized chemicals serve many specific functions beyond the basic life processes of growth, energy generation, and reproduction, they are referred to as "secondary metabolites". That is, they are secondary to the basic biochemical pathways possessed by both animals and plants that produce the enzymes, cofactors, and other chemicals that support the basic life functions common to all living organisms.

Since these secondary metabolites have evolved to possess biological activities that specifically benefit the plant, they are generally unique to plants—and are therefore foreign biologically active chemicals to members of the animal kingdom that consume the plants for nutritional benefit. Among the examples of highly toxic substances that are plant secondary metabolites are ricin, the rat poison (and anticoagulant medicine) warfarin, the convulsant strychnine, which has been used as a rodent and bird poison, the South American arrow poison curare, digitalis, nicotine, which was previously used as a pesticide but is no longer approved for this use due to its toxicity, and coniine (the toxic constituent of poison hemlock made famous by Socrates' death). Some of these chemicals are fatal to humans at amounts ranging from less than one-millionth of an ounce to a few thousandths of an ounce. The cereal crop sorghum contains specialized structures that produce the defensive compound dhurrin, which is hydrolyzed to highly toxic hydrogen cyanide in response to damage to the plant from pests. Young stressed seedlings may contain 30% dhurrin by weight, produced by a highly efficient complex of plant enzymes. The widely used pyrethroid insecticides were first discovered as the insecticidal constituents of chrysanthemums, which are members of the plant genus *Pyrethrum*. The effectiveness of these plant-derived pesticides has led to the synthesis of many additional synthetic chemical analogs that are now used as commercial pesticides. However, more important than examples of chemical constituents that are so toxic that they are not part of our food supply is our daily exposure to the many thousands of defensive chemicals with poorly characterized toxic potential that are exempted from safety testing by current regulatory guidelines meant to assure food and drug safety. These are constituents of the products that are preferentially sought by consumers who have the misconception that natural origin assures safety.

Many secondary metabolites have biological activities that we humans have exploited for our own benefit as medicinal drugs. Most of these are toxic at sufficient doses. Examples are the narcotic analgesics morphine and codeine, the anticholinergic drugs atropine and scopolamine, the heart failure drug digitalis, nicotine, the antimalarial drug quinine, numerous anticancer drugs including the taxanes, etoposide, and camptothecin, the gout treatment colchicine, and many others. Indeed the study of drug substances of natural origin is recognized as a scientific discipline and is termed pharmacognosy. Other biologically active metabolites have been, or are being, used as pesticides or dietary supplements. It has recently been estimated that the world market for plant extracts and isolated secondary metabolites exceeds $10 billion USD annually. An excellent in-depth discussion of plant secondary metabolites, including their role in plant defense and how biotechnology is being used to exploit their biological activities for human benefit, is available in a volume edited for Annual Plant Reviews by Michael Wink (1999; see reference list).

Since these defensive chemicals have evolved specifically to have biological activity, either noxious or toxic to deter predation or attractive to recruit insects or microbes that are beneficial to the plant, there is every reason to expect that their toxic potential should not differ from that of chemicals synthesized by humans to achieve the same purposes. However, because those synthesized by humans are required to be extensively tested for safety before use while those synthesized by the plant are not, it is highly likely that the natural plant-derived chemicals present the greater risk.

In fact, contrary to the belief of many people that "natural" plants are free of chemicals that might present a health risk, plants are an important source of exposure to a wide variety of naturally occurring and biologically active chemicals. This includes plant food products. Some people believe natural plants are actually free of "chemicals", and many think "synthetic" or "man-made" food constituents such as food additives and pesticide residues are the only potentially hazardous chemical constituents in our foods. We tend to view the world from our own human perspective, and as a result many have come to believe that plants must be safe and beneficial because they are a necessary source of nutrition. However, nature is not benign and plants didn't come into existence to provide nutritional benefit to humans. Rather, plants are complex organisms that have existed far longer than humans and have evolved sophisticated defensive and offensive mechanisms to deter and defeat their enemies. Like all living things, the well-being of a plant depends on obtaining the necessary food (nutrients) and water, and on defending itself from would-be predators and competitors that would either kill it and use it for its own food or compete with it for essential nutrients and water. Those enemies include microorganisms, insects, and animal predators that infect and consume the plants. We humans are one of those animal predators, and if viewed from the plant's perspective one of the smarter and therefore more dangerous ones.

The fact that traditional foods and "natural" botanical dietary supplements have generally been considered to be inherently safe has led to regulations governing the safety testing of these products that are far less rigorous than those governing products such as food additives, pesticides, and pharmaceutical products, which have been the focus of more concern. As a consequence, plant products considered to be traditional foods and botanical supplements are allowed to be sold without rigorous premarket safety testing whereas food additives, pesticides, and pharmaceutical products must be rigorously tested and the evidence of safety reviewed and approved by the responsible government regulatory body prior to sale. Many products are advertised as "organic" or "pesticide free", creating the impression that such products are safer because of the absence of toxic pesticides or chemical additives. But, is it an accurate assumption that such products are safer because they are not treated with pesticides during cultivation or with chemically synthesized preservatives to stabilize the final product?

Because plants are immobile and cannot run from predators or fight physically, they have evolved other methods of self-defense and manipulation of their environment. Some plants rely in part on thorns, surface barriers, or the ability to regrow damaged parts rapidly, but in general chemical warfare is their main method of defense against predators and diseases. It is the principal defense against the plants' main enemies: insects, fungi, nematodes, and animal predators. As any gardener can attest, all plants face formidable challenges from insect predators and diseases, and resistance to these challenges varies widely among different types and varieties of plants. In addition, plants use chemical signaling to attract favorable insect and animal species as well as to signal other plants of the need to respond to local predators. Plants synthesize many thousands of chemicals to perform these vital functions.

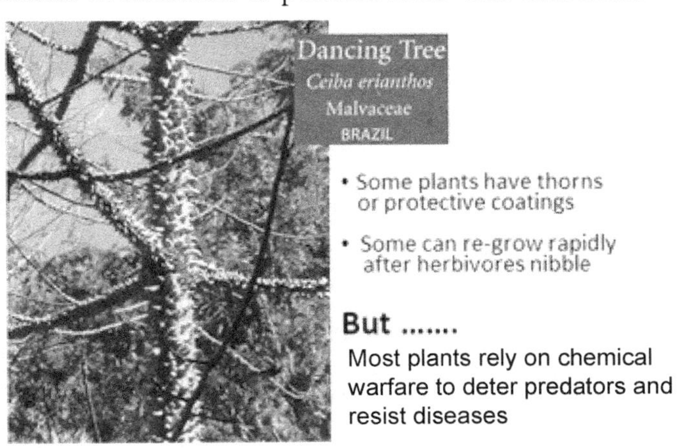

Since the very survival of plant species depends on their ability to resist, avoid, or compensate for attack by predators such as insects, fungi, nematodes, and herbivores, it is to be expected that the plant food products in stores either have been treated with commercial pesticides or fungicides, or have been selected to be insect and disease resistant (*i.e.*, selected to contain natural chemicals that protect them from predation and diseases).

Because synthetic pesticides are required to be intensively tested and the maximum residue levels are controlled to a very small fraction of that shown to cause any toxicity but organic crops contain uncharacterized and untested natural pesticides due to selective breeding for insect and disease resistance, one must seriously question the assumption that the latter are necessarily safer than conventionally produced products.

Even common food plants contain potentially toxic substances, such as the baby cucumber shown below at high magnification to reveal the poison sacks containing the bitter toxicants cucurbitacins that deter insect predators. Humans are smart enough to select as foods those plants that do not contain levels of secondary metabolites that cause *immediate* toxicity when consumed in normal dietary amounts and have learned to process the foods to reduce or eliminate acutely toxic components. However, effects such as delayed toxicities or the development of diseases that may require years to become manifest can usually be detected only if specific prospective studies are undertaken to identify them.

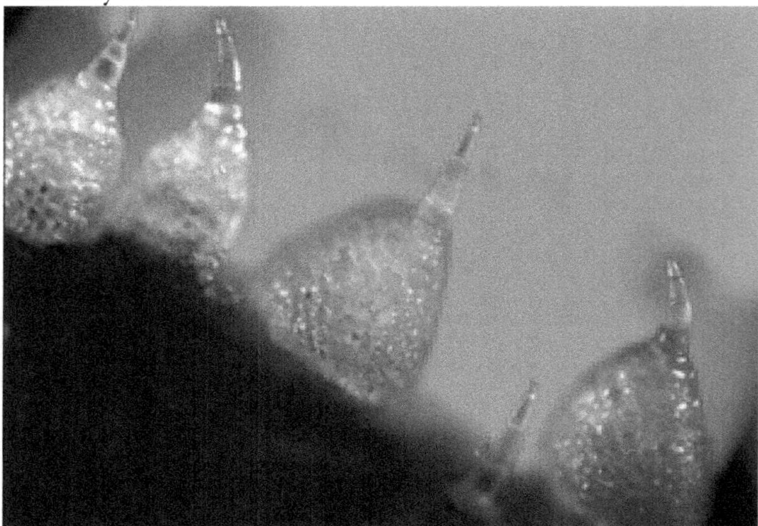

Figure 2.1: Surface of baby cucumber showing insect defense system
(From original color image by Robert Belliveau, Science 335: p. 525, 2012 with permission)

Studies have found that normal foods naturally contain substances that are capable of inducing effects such as genetic changes that could lead to delayed health effects such as the induction of cancer. For example, the careful studies of van der Hoeven *et al.* (1983) have shown that specific varieties of some common vegetables contain mutagens (chemicals that can damage DNA and cause genetic changes that can be passed from cell to cell or generation to generation). These investigators grew various strains of common vegetables side by side in identical plots so that environmental conditions and nutrient availability were the same for all the plants. They then evaluated extracts of the different cultivars to determine if they contained chemicals that damaged DNA and caused structural DNA changes that could be inherited—thereby modifying the function of the proteins whose structure was encoded by the DNA sequence. These studies used the same assay used to evaluate the mutagenic potential of new food additives, drugs, or pesticides before they are permitted to be marketed (foods that have a long history of use are not required to be tested in the same way as are food additives, new drugs, or pesticides). The studies showed that many of the cultivars contain mutagenic substances and that there is

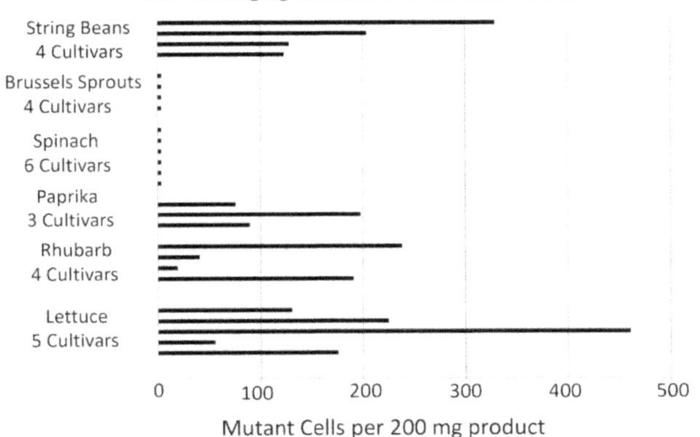

Figure 2.2: DNA-damaging substances in extracts of common food cultivars
Data are the number of mutant cells resulting from exposure to chemical extract from 200 mg (less than 1/100th of an ounce) of common food products (Figure drawn from the data of van der Hoeven *et al.*, J. Agric. Food Chem. 31: 1020-26, 1983)

considerable variation in the content of these substances among cultivars (see Figure 2.2).

This example is not to suggest that consumption of common vegetables is necessarily a health risk, but rather to emphasize that:

1. If similar mutagenic responses were induced by a food additive or a new pharmaceutical or pesticide under development, this would be a matter of regulatory concern that would require in-depth studies to determine the risk of mutagenic damage and subsequent disease under the conditions of proposed use. Indeed, many pharmaceutical companies have a policy of discontinuing development of potential drugs in certain classes when this type of response is discovered.

2. Applicable laws and regulatory policies are such that the dietary intake of mutagenic, and therefore potentially cancer-causing, substances from plant products is not generally evaluated—especially in the case of common foods that are considered to be safe by virtue of their long history of use.

This illustrates one of many important discrepancies in the overall regulatory structure for the safety assurance of marketed products. It also illustrates the general attitude of both average consumers and scientific regulatory authorities, who generally assume that common foods and botanical products are inherently safe but that chemically synthesized food additives, pharmaceuticals, or pesticides are potential health risks that require far more intense safety testing than the former, and often more extensively consumed, products—even to the extent of differently interpreting objective scientific data that show the same hazard signals in each case.

Because essentially all chemicals, and especially those with demonstrated biological activities, are toxic at some level of exposure, and because certain types of delayed toxicity (such as the induction of cancer, birth defects, or certain types of neurological disease) are not obvious unless specific studies are conducted to identify this potential, it is logical to ask why the biologically active chemicals synthesized by plants should not undergo the same standard of safety evaluation as do foreign chemicals such as pesticide residues or food additives. Is it logical to assume that those chemicals that happen to be made by plants, for the benefit of the plant, are necessarily safer than those chemicals made by man, to protect the plant for the benefit of man? Of course humans have selected agricultural plants that do not cause immediate acute toxicities when consumed at normal levels—but that does not necessarily protect against delayed or cumulative effects such as cancer, subtle neurological or immunological effects, or effects that occur only in susceptible individuals.

In this chapter, I invite the reader to reflect on these issues while considering the world from the plants' point of view. Consider the needs of the plant and the evolutionary forces that led to their capability to synthesize the chemicals that they produce. Plant enemies come in various sizes, from viruses, bacteria, molds, and small parasites to large predators capable of consuming an entire individual plant in a single encounter. Physical barriers such as bark, cuticles, or thorns play a role in keeping out microbial invaders and preventing predation by herbivores and a plant's ability to regrow allows recovery from moderate predation—however, chemical warfare is the most widely used among the defense mechanisms available to plants.

The evolution of the ability to synthesize endogenous chemicals that are toxic to predators or competitors, that inhibit their growth, or that deter unwanted species through noxious taste or odor is a common characteristic of plants and also of microorganisms. Bacteria make antibiotics when growth conditions are poor and they go dormant, in order to kill or inhibit the growth of competitive organisms. Of course everyone knows the story of Fleming's discovery of penicillin, which is an antibacterial product of the *Penicillium* mold. These microbiocidal chemicals have generally evolved to be directed against other competitive microorganisms, but they may also be toxic to higher organisms. For example, botulinum toxin, produced by the bacterium *Clostridium botulinum*, is one of the most acutely lethal toxins known. It has been estimated that approximately two pounds of this toxin could paralyze or kill every human on the planet! Like microbes, plants have also developed effective means of chemical warfare against harmful organisms, as well as chemical manipulation of organisms that they "wish" to attract or repel. Evolutionary pressure has facilitated the development in plants of the ability to synthesize the vast array of secondary metabolites that allow them to deter predation, protect against infective organisms, attract beneficial insects and other species, and in general to control the behavior of other living organisms in their environment. These chemicals are often stored in high concentrations in particular areas of the plant, and their synthesis may be induced in response to damage caused by a predator or pathogen. For example, volatile compounds from damaged chrysanthemum plants stimulate the synthesis of pyrethrin insecticides in neighboring plants. The role of secondary metabolites as deterrents to predation and as attractants to beneficial species is well-known, and the continued use of naturally derived pesticides and their synthetic analogs attests to their importance and effectiveness.

The influence of plants on other organisms by means of chemical interactions is known as allelopathy, and allelochemicals are the secondary metabolites that have detrimental or beneficial effects on target organisms. Allelopathy is common in many plants and has been relatively intensively studied in trees, desert shrubs, rice, and other agricultural crops. Laboratory studies have shown many cases of inhibitory effects of plant extracts, plant components, or specific chemicals derived from plants on seed germination and growth of other plant species. Negative allelopathic effects (growth suppression) by plants on plant species that compete for space, nutrients, and water is particularly notable among desert plants, where competition for water and nutrients is most intense. Desert plants often use both physical defense in the form of thorns and thick protective coats to deter predators and also deploy chemicals that inhibit the growth of other plants. Plant-plant chemical interactions are often complex and involve interactions with the environment, nutrient supply, and stress factors. Allelopathic effects are well-known to agricultural scientists and knowledgeable gardeners. A discussion of these issues in Wikipedia provides references for further reading (http://wikipedia.org/wiki/Allelopathy).

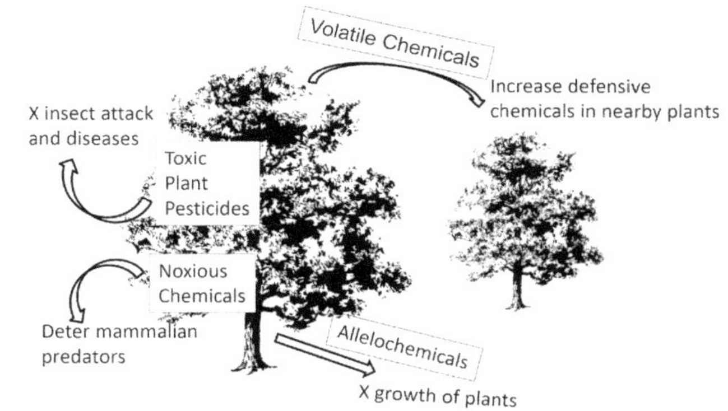

Figure 2.3: *Types of plant chemical defenses*

Plants do not have the same type of immune systems as do animals to protect them from attack by pathogens or predators, but they do have specialized biochemical pathways that can recognize and respond to pathogen- or predator-induced physical damage caused by animals or insects, stress, or attack by pathogens. Chemicals known as oxylipins or octadecanoids, derived from linoleic or α-linolenic acids, are involved in these responses. Among these oxylipins, jasmonates are an especially important class of chemicals involved in plant responses to wounding. These chemicals are important signals that activate genes that code for defensive chemicals or macromolecules, compounds that discourage consumption due to offensive taste or bitterness, or toxic chemicals that deter insect herbivores and in effect "immunize" the plant against further attack.

Volatile jasmonate derivatives also serve as aerial defenses by deterring herbivorous species, attracting predators of the plant herbivores, and even inducing defense responses in nearby plants. See the appended reading list for more information on the sophisticated defenses that have evolved in plants. In order to survive and thrive without mobility in a competitive and hostile world, plants, of necessity, have become masters of chemical defense and chemical warfare!

An interesting example that illustrates the sophistication of this evolutionary defensive process is the evolution of carnivorous plants such as the Venus flytrap. The flytrap has evolved the ability to use the jasmonate chemical-signaling pathway just described, which was originally evolved to protect itself against insects and harmful microorganisms, to "turn the tables" and digest and consume insects—thereby making the plant the predator. Such plants have evolved the ability to use this same pathway to produce enzymes that destroy components of insects or microbes such as insect chitin—thus allowing the plant to digest and absorb the insects as food. The evolution of these carnivorous plants exemplifies the age-old dictum that offense is the best defense, by turning would-be predators into a food source for the plant!

So complex is this ongoing chemical warfare that the chemical signals that have evolved in one species of plant for its own benefit are sometimes highjacked by competitive species and used against the originator of the signaling molecules. One notable example of this is the way the parasitic witchweed (Strigia) plant attacks crops such as rice, corn, millet, cotton, and sorghum. Witchweed is a worldwide agricultural problem. It is estimated that only one species of witchweed causes about $10 billion in crop losses in Africa alone. An outbreak in the Carolinas in the U.S. in the 1950s spurred an extensive eradication program and also generated the research that led to an understanding of how these parasitic plants attack and severely damage crop plants. The crop plants make chemicals called strigolactones that act as hormonal signals that stimulate plant growth and also stimulate the growth of soil fungi that form symbiotic connections with the host plants. Witchweed effectively parasitizes the crop plants by producing huge numbers of seeds (up to 100,000 per plant) that lie dormant until a vulnerable host plant begins to grow nearby. The witchweed seeds sense the presence of the strigolactones produced by the emerging crop plants and then germinate and send out roots that penetrate the host plant's root and suck out the nutrients.

Of course the fact that plants contain so many biologically active chemicals, and that some of these have unpleasant taste or odor or can produce illness when consumed, does not mean that consumption of plant foods should be avoided. On the contrary, we depend on plants for nutrition and survival. It must be appreciated that virtually all chemicals have the potential to cause adverse effects at some extremely high dose, and that health risks can only be evaluated by considering effects as a function of the level of exposure. It cannot be assumed that the presence of chemicals that have the potential to cause adverse health effects at high levels of exposure are necessarily bad at those levels of exposure that occur under actual conditions of use. Many chemicals have no effect, and some have beneficial effects, at low to moderate levels of exposure and almost all have adverse effects at exaggerated exposure levels. Only by understanding the potential for specific forms of toxicity at higher doses and then evaluating the relationship of that knowledge to an understanding of the effects at levels normally consumed can health risks and benefits be evaluated properly. In other words, it is not useful to attempt to choose products based on a qualitative classification of a chemical that it contains as good *vs.* bad, or toxic *vs.* nontoxic, because health risks and health benefits depend on the level of exposure and different effects may be expressed at different levels of exposure. As has been pointed out, it would be a very poor health choice to decide to filter the oxygen out of the air we breathe because extended exposure to pure or hyperbaric oxygen poses health risks and can result in death. Systematic study and control of product and chemical safety consists of three phases: 1) hazard assessment, in which *potential* toxicities are determined by using exaggerated exposures high enough to induce adverse effects; 2) risk assessment, in which the specific quantitative risk of an adverse effect at actual expected levels of exposure in real-life situations is evaluated; and 3) risk management, in which specific procedures and safety margins are established that prevent harmful effects under conditions of actual use.

Humans, of course, are highly intelligent and have long used domestication strategies to select those plants that can be consumed without obvious toxic consequences. We also employ production and processing methods that minimize or eliminate exposure to undesirable chemical constituents. These strategies have enabled us to cultivate plants that meet our nutritional needs in spite of the evolutionary pressure on plants to synthesize defensive chemicals that may in some cases be noxious or toxic to man. The classic book on the development of human civilization by Jared Diamond, *Guns, Germs, and Steel* (1999), emphasizes the importance of domestication of wild plants and the resultant advantages of crop food production as a key element in the development of successful civilizations. Both plants and animals are modified when domesticated, both by selection of those species and individuals with desirable characteristics and also through genetic modification by selective breeding of those variants with characteristics desirable by the human domesticators. According to Diamond, only about 200 of the many thousands of wild plants have been domesticated for human food consumption and only 12 species account for approximately 80% of the world food production—wheat, corn, rice, barley, sorghum, soybean, potato, cassava (manioc), sweet potato, sugar cane, sugar beet, and banana.

Numerous examples could be cited to illustrate how we have domesticated specific varieties of agricultural plants and manipulated their properties through selective breeding so that they lack the undesirable characteristics of their wild ancestors. A recent example that has appeared in the prestigious journal *Science* is that of the plant family *Cucurbitaceae*, which includes cucumber, melons, squash, pumpkin, and watermelon. The wild ancestors of these plants contain bitter triterpenes called cucurbitacins in high concentration, making them extremely bitter. In the cucumber these chemicals are concentrated in trichomes, which are the fuzzy coat on the surface of the cucumber. As shown in Figure 2.1, at high magnification this fuzzy coat is in fact revealed to be a layer of bulbous containers for these bitter-tasting and toxic chemicals that are tipped with a point that can pierce the mouths of small predators. A series of genetic and biochemical studies has shown that domestication practices have greatly reduced the concentration of these bitter chemicals in the edible parts of this family of food plants through selection of strains that contain genetic elements that suppress the synthesis of the bitter components (Shang *et al.*, 2014). This example is typical of the continuing balance between the evolutionary need of plants to produce secondary metabolites that provide defense and attract beneficial organisms and humans' efforts to select and manipulate for cultivation as food sources plants that have a chemical content that is a desirable balance of pest resistance during cultivation and acceptable taste and nontoxic characteristics in the consumed product. In other words, plants have evolved the ability to synthesize naturally occurring pest deterrents and pesticides and humans have been modifying the content of these chemicals for millennia though selective cultivation practices and selective breeding that result in genetic characteristics that determine a chemical composition compatible with their use as a food source. In fact, the selective cultivation and breeding practices can be thought of as a form of genetic engineering, because, just as direct genetic modification of the DNA in genetically engineered plants changes the genetic makeup of the plant and thereby modifies its chemical composition, these common agricultural practices of selective breeding and selective cultivation also result in plants that are genetically different, and that have a different chemical composition, from the wild species that have been domesticated.

These selective practices are used both for the purpose of reducing the content of objectionable or toxic chemicals, as in the *Cucurbitaceae* example above, or to increase the content of natural pest deterrents, as in the selection of pest- and disease-resistant plants by organic farmers who don't wish to use man-made pesticides. As will be discussed in a subsequent chapter on the regulations that apply to food safety assurance, there is no general requirement to prospectively evaluate the safety of the elevated levels of secondary metabolites in new cultivars of pest-resistant plants, whereas extensive safety testing would be required in the case of a new pesticide added by man that results in a residue in the edible product. Thus, evaluation of the latter, but not the former, will include studies to examine potential delayed and low-frequency, but serious, health effects that would not be apparent without specific testing.

It is also relevant to note that animals have evolved a complex set of metabolic capabilities that enable them to detoxify and excrete foreign chemical substances such as plant secondary metabolites. The enzymes involved in these metabolic detoxification pathways undoubtedly evolved to enable animals to consume a wide variety of plant food sources that contained chemicals that would otherwise be toxic. Although complex, one general feature of these detoxification systems is the conversion of chemicals from forms that are accumulated in the body to metabolically altered forms with characteristics that facilitate their excretion from the body. Just as many of the plant secondary metabolites that serve specific defensive functions for the plant are specific to the plant kingdom, many of these detoxification enzymes are specific to the animal kingdom. Without these detoxification mechanisms, many of the constituents to which we are exposed on a daily basis would accumulate to toxic levels. Thus, nature's evolutionary forces have created a balance, whereby plants have developed one set of biochemical properties that allows them to successfully grow and compete without the advantage of mobility, and animals, including humans, have developed biochemical characteristics that protect them from harmful effects of the chemicals in plants and that allow them to derive nutritional benefit from plants by protecting themselves against plant metabolites that would otherwise be toxic. Notably, the mammalian detoxification enzymes have very general specificity and also function to metabolize and detoxify man-made industrial chemicals, pharmaceutical drugs, synthetic pesticides, and other chemicals that we ingest or to which we are exposed in our environment.

Taste and odor are additional factors that relate to this competition between plants and animals. It appears that natural selection among foraging animals favors those that perceive the taste and odor of nutritious and nontoxic plants as favorable and those of toxic plants as noxious. Thus natural selection during evolution has been proposed to lead to a taste and odor system in which it is the most nutritionally beneficial and healthful food sources that are perceived as attractive, and those that are toxic or that produce digestive problems are perceived as noxious. In support of this idea, studies of acceptance-rejection reflexes across a wide phylogenetic range of organisms and development stages have shown that these reflexes are located in the brainstem and are not affected by the loss of neural tissue in the areas of the brain associated with higher functions—and are therefore innate to the most basic neural functions of the brain. This suggests that these characteristics are a basic feature of the animal kingdom and that they have been conserved through evolution due to their importance to survival and competition for resources. Perhaps humans have now evolved to the point that rational scientific evaluation of the effects of the plant-derived chemicals to which we are exposed can begin to play an equally, or more, important role in our food choices, but sensory-based food choices certainly continue to influence our dietary choices and are expected to continue to play an important role in the balance of plant-animal competition in lower organisms.

In summary, plants contain a vast array of secondary metabolites that often have biological activity in other organisms, including humans. Agricultural practices continually modify the content of these chemicals in the plants that are selected and bred for food production. In addition to their presence in food products, some of these chemicals have been developed as commercial pharmaceutical products and others are contained in plant products, extracts, or concentrates sold as dietary supplements. The safety of these chemicals should be considered objectively in the context of our overall exposure to environmental chemicals. The assumptions that chemicals produced naturally by plants are necessarily innocuous and that man-made food additives and pesticide residues are necessarily harmful at the levels present in food products are not accurate. The safety of each chemical, or class of chemicals, whether natural or man-made, should be evaluated objectively by the same standards and should be based on the development of a scientific understanding of the potential for specific forms of toxicity (*i.e.*, a formal hazard assessment) and the use of that knowledge to define the adverse and beneficial effects at levels normally consumed (*i.e.*, a risk assessment). Current requirements for the safety evaluation of both plant-derived and man-made products vary widely and are the subject of subsequent chapters.

Chapter 3
Toxic Effects and Their Causes Can Be Hard to Identify: Why Serious Toxicities Often Escape Identification

Among the important misconceptions that underpin the natural mistake is the belief that the long history of use of many traditional herbal products without known deleterious effects provides assurance of their safety. The same reasoning with respect to organic food products and basic conventional foods underpins the current regulatory structure that requires stringent safety testing of chemical additives, colorants, and pesticide residues before a product can be sold but does not require that naturally occurring food products, their constituents, or botanical supplements be tested in the same way. Some of the reasons why a history of use is not adequate evidence of safety have already been mentioned and the well-documented cases that follow highlight some of the difficulties encountered in identifying toxicities and in establishing the causative factor once the occurrence of toxicity has been recognized. These cases illustrate that serious human toxicities often go unrecognized for extended periods. It is a virtual certainty that many other cases of adverse health effects remain unidentified. Natural is not always safe, causative agents are not easy to identify, and widespread risk may not be obvious. After considering these cases, the value of prospective safety evaluation should be evident.

Given the many natural plant products, including common food plants, that have been identified as being toxic at certain stages of development, having toxic parts, or that are toxic unless processed, it is not surprising that toxicities from plant products have occurred. No attempt will be made to catalog known toxic plants here, but examples are numerous. For example, one Wikipedia article on toxic plants lists more than 100 species and genera of plants known to be toxic to humans and/or animals, fifteen of which are common food plants (http://en.wikipedia. org/wiki/List_of_poisonous_plants). Poisonous constituents of common foods include cyanogenic (cyanide-forming) glycosides (sugar or carbohydrate conjugates) that occur in peach, plum, almond, cherry, and apricot seeds and leaves, as well as in lima beans and cassava roots and leaves, phytohemagglutinins in kidney beans, various alkaloids, glycoalkaloids, oxalic acid, urushiol, myristicin, glucosinolates, and many other chemicals in various plant foodstuffs. Most of these are acutely toxic and so their toxicity is easy to identify because toxicity develops relatively rapidly after ingestion and the association of the toxic outcome with the exposure is therefore obvious. We have learned to select, process, and prepare the foods containing these acutely toxic substances in a manner that allows their consumption without the development of acute toxicities in most cases. Even so, many cases of toxicity from well-characterized acutely toxic products or contaminants still occur. For example, almost 1000 cases of poisoning associated with plants containing belladonna alkaloids, which are well-known to cause a form of toxicity called anticholinergic syndrome, were reported to poison control centers in the U.S. in a single year (CDC Morbidity and Mortality Weekly Reports, 1995). In the U.S., this type of toxicity is most often due to contamination with one of the many plants that contain belladonna alkaloids and in other parts of the world may result from improper preparation of food plants such as lupin that are known to contain this class of alkaloids.

Far more difficult to identify are toxicities that do not occur immediately after exposure, that occur only in sensitive individuals, or that occur as a result of an interaction with a second factor. These often remain undetected for extended periods even when the toxicity is extremely serious, debilitating, or lethal. The examples of such human toxicities that follow each illustrate a different situation that allowed a severe and/or life-threatening toxicity to remain unrecognized for a considerable period before eventually being traced to an exposure to a particular food, dietary supplement, or medicinal drug. They also show that the eventual discovery of such effects is often a matter of chance.

These examples are not meant to suggest that natural products, in general, are inherently less safe than conventional ones, or to generalize about the safety of either natural or man-made chemicals. Rather, the examples are meant 1) to show that such generalizations are not meaningful because each class contains both deleterious and beneficial chemicals, and 2) to emphasize that safety assurance of any product can only be achieved by careful and comprehensive safety studies in conjunction with production controls and identity standards that assure consistent well-characterized products free of undesirable impurities. With this in mind, these examples highlight the difficulty of identifying the causes of even serious health effects and illustrate the necessity of systematic premarket safety testing of all product classes if safety is to be assured. It should also become evident that a long history of use without apparent adverse effects provides only assurance of a lack of marked *acute* toxicity, but does not rule out serious or even lethal toxicities that require a period of time after exposure to develop, that occur only in certain individuals with susceptibility factors, that result from interaction with other agents, or that are dependent on a specific genetic defect or characteristic.

The *Aristolochia* Story: Identification of the cause of serious toxicity is often difficult even when strong clues are present

The *Aristolochia* story, in which the causative agent of the severe kidney disease now known as aristolochic acid nephropathy (AAN) was traced to herbal preparations or dietary contamination with components of plants of the genus *Aristolochia,* is an example that illustrates how much focused research effort is needed to establish causality of a severe toxicity even when there is strong evidence that the effect must be due to a specific exposure in a defined group of individuals. In spite of causing severe kidney toxicity and an extremely high rate of cancer in the kidney and urinary tract, only the "lucky" occurrence of two situations led to identification of the cause of a serious disease and brought to light the toxic properties of the widely used herbal preparations that contain these plant toxicants.

Aristolochia is a genus of plants containing species that have been used for hundreds, or perhaps thousands, of years as herbal remedies. Until recently, these herbal products were considered to be beneficial and safe. Then two separate lines of scientific investigation, both spurred by unusual circumstances, demonstrated the toxic potential of certain chemicals in these plants. Had these two unusual events not occurred, the very serious worldwide health risk posed by the widespread use of these herbs would almost certainly still be unknown.

The first of these events was the recognition of an unusual kidney disease that occurred in very specific small rural areas along the Danube River in the Balkan area that now includes Bosnia, Bulgaria, Croatia, Romania, and Serbia. This kidney disease was named Balkan endemic nephropathy, or BEN. Because this severe kidney disease occurred only in very specific rural areas and did not occur in similar nearby villages, it was suspected that it was caused by exposure to some toxic agent in the environment, in the food, or in water. This disease was known as early as the 1920s but was not described as a specific disease in the medical literature until 1956 by the Bulgarian nephrologist Yoto Tanchev and coworkers. At least 25,000 individuals in the rural affected areas are believed to have suffered from this disease. Although extensive studies were undertaken to identify the causative agent during the next 50 years, the cause remained unknown until a tragic event occurred in Brussels, Belgium, in the early 1990s that provided a clue that pointed to the causative agent. In the Brussels disaster, a Chinese herb containing a preparation from the plant *Aristolochia fangchi* was mistakenly used in an herbal weight loss product and led to the development of severe kidney damage in more than 100 people. The disease in the Brussels case was originally referred to as Chinese herbal nephropathy, or CHN. Because the patients from this severe and unusual nephropathy were concentrated in one clinic, the cluster of toxicity was recognized. Had the background prevalence of this specific type of kidney pathology been higher and had the patients been dispersed among many different clinics, perhaps even such a severe toxicity would have gone unrecognized. Follow-up studies of these patients showed that urothelial cancer rates in those subjects with severe nephropathy were extraordinarily high—40 to 46% of the patients with late-stage nephropathy caused by exposure to *Aristolochia* developed this type of cancer.

The finding of such a severe human toxicity and high carcinogenic activity led to extensive laboratory animal studies and concurrent studies of the poisoning victims in Belgium. These studies resulted in the identification of the causative agent as the herbal preparation of *Aristolochia fangchi*. The laboratory studies established that aristolochic acid, present in this herb, was a potent renal carcinogen and caused characteristic chemical modification of the DNA (DNA adducts) in the affected kidneys. The type of kidney pathology that occurred in the poisoning incident in Belgium was recognized as being very similar, if not identical, to that in the local endemic kidney disease in the Balkan area. This, in turn, led to investigations of the possibility that the Balkan kidney disease might be caused by either similar herbal preparations used in the affected Balkan populations or by contamination of the food supply with *Aristolochia* plants or plant components. After intensive studies of the affected population and of the biological basis of the severe kidney toxicity in patients with Balkan endemic nephropathy, it was demonstrated that the same chemical identified as the causative agent of the kidney toxicity in the incident in Belgium, aristolochic acid (and possibly closely related chemicals in the same plants), occurs in the seeds of *Aristolochia* plants that grow in wheat fields in the Balkan region. Studies showed that contamination of fields with *Aristolochia* was correlated with the occurrence of BEN, and that seeds containing aristolochic acid and related chemicals became mixed with the wheat upon harvest and contaminated the wheat and wheat flour. Analysis of specific DNA adducts in the tumors and kidneys of affected patients and of laboratory animals showed that exposure to aristolochic acid results in the same specific "signature" of chemical DNA adducts described above in both patients and laboratory animals exposed to aristolochic acid. Sufficient exposure to aristolochic acid and related chemicals from *Aristolochia* plants has thus been shown to lead to kidney and urinary tract cancers in both laboratory animals and in the patients suffering from the Balkan kidney disease and the so-called Chinese herbal nephropathy. Thus, Chinese herbal (or herbs) nephropathy and Balkan endemic nephropathy are now considered to be the same disease, which has been given the more general name of aristolochic acid nephropathy.

It is now clearly understood that *Aristolochia* species containing aristolochic acid are highly toxic to the kidney and are potent human renal carcinogens. Of critical importance, this work has led to the realization that many herbal products containing aristolochic acid have long been used in China and other Asian countries and that such products are sold *via* the internet in the United States and other countries. These herbal products contain this same toxic ingredient and appear to present a serious world-wide health risk (*e.g.,* Debelle *et al.,* 2008).   Only now are the potential health consequences of these uses being investigated. Were it not for the unfortunate cases of the Brussels poisoning incident and the concentration of severe cases of *Aristolochia* poi-soning in the Balkan area, this widespread risk associated with other herbal products would likely still be unrecognized.

Aristolochic acid and plants containing aristolochic acid are now classified by the International Agency for Research on Cancer, the recognized international authority that evaluates and classifies cancer-causing agents, as "known to be carcino-genic to humans" (Group 1, the highest possible classification). Although Chinese herbs nephropathy (CHN) was originally identified in the outbreak of nephropathy in Belgium, additional cases have now been reported in France, Spain, Japan, the United Kingdom, and Taiwan. Many traditional Chinese herbal medi-cines still contain *Aristolochia* species, and it is very likely that the use of these medicines has caused, and is continuing to cause, a large number of unrecognized *Aristolochia*-related cases of kidney toxicity and urinary tract cancer worldwide.

This story illustrates the difficulty of identifying caus-ative agents even when exposures result in severe toxicity and are localized to very specific populations. When adverse health effects are less severe, are not concentrated in a specific small population, when the effects also occur spontaneously in the general population, and when there is a significant time inter-val between exposure and manifestation of the resultant toxicity or disease, it is very difficult to identify even the fact that there is an adverse effect, let alone identify the causative agent. The unique characteristics of Balkan endemic neuropathy, including its highly localized occurrence, specific characteristics of kidney and urinary tract damage, the unusually high incidence of upper urinary tract cancers, combined with the occurrence of affected villages located in close proximity to unaffected ones—and with a spatial distribution of the disease that has remained relatively unchanged with time—would be expected to make identification of the causative agent unusually easy. Nonetheless, the cause of this disease remained unknown despite 50 years of scientific study.

It is noteworthy that the initial suspected causes of this disease included viruses, exposure to chemicals believed to have leached from nearby coal deposits, mold contamination of the food supply resulting in exposure to mold toxins such as ochratoxin A, selenium deficiency, and exposure to heavy metals. These hypotheses originated, of course, from the knowledge of specific toxic agents with properties that might cause the types of pathology observed. Contamination with a plant constituent was not initially suspected as a potential cause of this disease. After all, scientists are human and are led to explore that which is most familiar to them.

This case illustrates how even very toxic dietary constituents that are used for extended periods at doses that cause severe harm can remain undetected unless carefully controlled scientific investigations are undertaken to identify the harmful effect, or unless chance events bring the problem to light. Even when a specific toxic syndrome is recognized, years of research may be required to identify the causative agent. It also illustrates that severe or fatal human poisoning may occur from commonly occurring plants thought to be harmless. Prospective studies designed to identify potential toxicities in combination with scientific assessment of the risks associated with the degree of exposure that occurs with actual product use are necessary to provide assurance of product safety prior to the occurrence of significant disease and suffering. In the absence of such systematic safety testing it is clearly inappropriate to conclude that a product is safe just because there is a long history of use in the absence of recognized adverse effects.

Ephedra: A long history of use as a medicinal agent and dietary supplement does not guarantee safety

Preparations of the *Ephedra sinica* plant or other species of the *Ephedra* genus have a long history of use as medicinal preparations, dietary supplements, and tea. In China, where ephedra has been used for millennia in medicinal preparations, it is referred to as ma huang. Ephedra contains many bioactive chemicals, including the alkaloids ephedrine and pseudoephedrine. It has been widely used as a weight loss aid and as a performance-enhancing drug by athletes. It increases metabolism, raises blood pressure, increases heart rate, and increases body temperature. As a dietary supplement, ephedra is regulated under the DSHEA, which, as has been noted, does not require premarket safety testing or defined quality and purity standards.

As the use of ephedra in the United States grew more widespread, reports of adverse effects accumulated, and increased attention was focused on the risks associated with its use. Studies then uncovered an association with heart attack, stroke, and sudden cardiac death. Analyses of commercial ephedra products showed major variations in the content of ephedrine alkaloid levels, even within the same brand. Between 1995 and 1997, the FDA received more than 900 reports of possible ephedra toxicity, including serious adverse events such as stroke, heart attack, and sudden death in 37 cases. Other effects included dizziness, trembling, headache, insomnia, perspiration, dehydration, vomiting, and hyperthermia. As a result of these risks, in 1997 the FDA proposed a ban on products containing 8 mg or more ephedrine alkaloid as well as stricter labeling requirements including disclosure of the risk of heart attack, stroke, or death. In response to this proposal, the supplement industry commissioned a scientific review by a private consulting firm that concluded that ephedra was safe. An Ephedra Education Council, a public relations group, was created to oppose the proposed FDA action. The events surrounding the industry response and the eventual FDA ban are summarized in a Wikipedia article on ephedra, with references (Wikipedia, 2016).

Between 1997 and 2000, the rebuttals to the FDA claims of health risk by the Ephedra Education Council, other industry lobbying, and questioning of the scientific basis of the FDA position by Senators Hatch and Harkin (who sponsored the DSHEA legislation) led to withdrawal of the proposed labeling changes and restrictions by the FDA. However, evidence of severe adverse reactions and death continued to mount. This included a review in the *New England Journal of Medicine* that reported cases of sudden cardiac death or severe disability in young adults using ephedra. Also, the Department of Justice mandated the release of more than 15,000 reports of ephedra-related adverse events, including deaths, which had been withheld by Metabolife, a major manufacturer of ephedra supplements. Perhaps of most consequence, ephedra use was associated with the deaths of two prominent athletes: Minnesota Vikings lineman Korey Stringer in 2001 and Baltimore Orioles pitcher Steve Bechler in 2003. According to an article in the *Los Angeles Times* (March 5, 2003), Senator Orrin Hatch, who had helped block the FDA's earlier attempts to regulate ephedra, stated after these new findings and reports that it was obvious that problems existed and referred to the FDA action to regulate ephedra as "long overdue". Finally, on April 12, 2004, the FDA issued a final rule banning the sale of ephedra-containing dietary supplements.

After the FDA ban, legal challenges to the ban continued for years. Nutraceutical Corporation claimed that the FDA had exceeded the authority allowed under the Dietary Supplement Health and Education Act and the US District Court for Utah ruled that it had not been proven that low doses of ephedra were unsafe. This ruling allowed the sale of ephedra in Utah and therefore called into question whether sales in other states could be stopped. This ruling was appealed and in 2006 the U.S. Court of Appeals in Denver upheld the FDA's ban on ephedra sales, concluding that the FDA had documented unreasonable risk from ephedra use. Nutraceutical Corporation then filed a request with the Supreme Court asking for a review of the lower court decision upholding the ban, but in 2007 the Supreme Court refused to hear this petition. Thus, the sale of ephedra-containing supplements remains prohibited in the United States.

This case illustrates several important points. First, the requirements for the safety evaluation of dietary supplements under DSHEA are extremely lax. Because premarket testing is not required before marketing dietary supplements, ephedra products were sold and used extensively prior to recognition of the health risks associated with its use. When extensive reports of adverse health effects accumulated, documentation of the relationship between ephedra use and the adverse effects was initially difficult because 1) the lack of a requirement for systematic premarket investigation and of controlled clinical trials meant that there was no coherent body of essential safety studies on which to base regulatory action; 2) unlike the case of pharmaceutical agents, in which the company selling the product must prove safety before the product is sold, the DSHEA law places the burden of proof of harm on the FDA before it is permitted to take action; and 3) the lack of requirements for standardized purity and identity resulted in a situation with a wide variation of bioactive alkaloids in different preparations, even those from the same manufacturer. Thus, much time was needed to assemble studies that were in many cases not exactly comparable in terms of either experimental design or of the chemical content of the products studied. This leaves considerable latitude for manufacturers to challenge the validity of scientific conclusions, and, with the burden of proof of harm on the regulatory agency that has not conducted the studies, FDA actions were left open to scientific and legal challenges. Both of these occurred and resulted in substantial delay in finally removing these dangerous and poorly controlled products from the market.

Finally, this case illustrates not only the difficulty of conclusively proving serious toxicities, even heart attack, stroke, and death, but highlights the barriers that the FDA faces when attempting to enforce controls on the sale of harmful supplements.

Fen-Phen: Serious and widespread toxicity can be missed even when a specific adverse event reporting system is in place

Although this case involves a drug product, it is included because it illustrates that even when an established adverse event reporting system is in place, as is the case with prescription drugs and dietary supplements, serious toxicities can still fail to be recognized. Fen-Phen is a nickname given to the combination of the two drugs fenfluramine and phentermine, which were widely prescribed in a combination treatment for obesity in the early 1990s. Although approved separately as anorectic agents by the FDA, the combination was not FDA-approved. Nonetheless, the use of the combination became widespread when it was found that lower doses of each could be used when the drugs were used in combination. It was thought that the lower doses would result in fewer side effects and improved patient tolerance. It is noteworthy that drugs must be tested and shown to be effective and safe when used in specific dosage regimens before they are approved by the FDA for sale for specific therapeutic indications, but that physicians have the latitude to prescribe drugs, or combinations of drugs, for therapeutic indications other than the specific indication for which they are FDA-approved. Thus, the use of the combination Fen-Phen treatment is similar to the use of many herbal supplements, in that this specific use and dosage regimen had not undergone the usual premarket testing required of approved drug products. It has been estimated that more than 18 million prescriptions for this combination were issued in 1996, the year before the occurrence of severe heart valve defects were found to be associated with the use of this drug combination.

In 1997 it was reported by a group of clinicians in the Rochester, Minnesota, area that they had recognized 24 cases of an unusual heart valve defect in women of an average age of 44 who had received, or were receiving, Fen-Phen for weight loss (Connolly *et al.*, 1997). These women, who had no previous history of cardiac disease, had heart murmurs, shortness of breath, congestive heart failure, edema, or other cardiac symptoms. Follow-up studies of these patients established that they all had abnormal leaky heart valves. The characteristics of the valve defects were unusual and were recognized to be similar to those caused by a rare cancerous tumor that secretes the chemical mediator serotonin. This astute group of physicians recognized that this cluster of extremely serious heart valve abnormalities was likely due to the Fen-Phen treatment regimen that was common to all the patients. They also noted that the similarity of the defects to those that occur in the rare carcinoid syndrome suggested that the mechanism was likely mediated by the effect of the combination of the two drugs on serotonin sensitivity or serotonin concentration modification because fenfluramine is known to affect serotonin metabolism and phentermine interferes with the clearance of serotonin by the lung.

An important feature of this case is that in the case of prescription drugs such as these, the FDA has in place an adverse event reporting system designed to detect drug-related toxicities. Physicians and patients are asked to report all unusual findings that might be related to drug treatments, and the FDA routinely reviews these reports to identify unsuspected toxicities that may not have been recognized during the drug development process. In spite of this well-established reporting system, this system failed to identify this serious drug-related toxicity until the astute observation of a team of physicians recognized that they were seeing a pattern of unusual cardiac toxicity in patients using this weight loss regimen. The report of this team of physicians was made public on July 8, 1997, more than a month before the official publication appeared in the *New England Journal of Medicine* on August 28, 1997. Following the public release of this information, the FDA sent letters to approximately 700,000 U.S. health care practitioners and institutions requesting information on similar patients. The FDA then received 120 additional reports of patients with similar effects.

Of more importance than these additional reports, recognition by physicians that symptoms of such valve defects usually don't appear until relatively advanced damage has occurred led to the conduct of five independent studies of patients who had received treatment with fenfluramine or dexfenfluramine with or without phentermine but who had no obvious history of cardiac disease or cardiac symptoms. These five studies all obtained similar findings using echocardiography and showed that 30-38% of the patients surveyed who did not have symptoms had measurable heart valve defects. This is an extraordinarily high frequency. Considering that more than 18 million prescriptions per year were being issued when this effect was finally discovered, the medical consequences were extremely extensive. As a result of these findings, the FDA requested voluntary withdrawal of fenfluramine and dexfenfluramine from the market. On September 15, 1997, less than one month after the formal publication of the initial findings at the Mayo clinic in the *New England Journal of Medicine* and slightly more than two months after the first public announcement of the initial observations, the manufacturers and the FDA announced the withdrawal of these drugs.

This case illustrates that even when prospective safety studies are conducted on the responsible agents and when a specific adverse event reporting system that is designed to detect unsuspected exposure-related toxicity is in place, extremely serious and widespread toxicities can remain undetected. Keeping in mind that prescription drugs such as fenfluramine and dexfenfluramine are the most thoroughly studied of the product classes under discussion, and that physicians are encouraged to be alert for and to report suspected drug exposure-related toxicities within a system subject to continuous monitoring by the FDA, how can one cite as assurance of safety "a long history of use" of those classes of products that can be sold without prospective safety assessment studies and with no stringent product identity and production standards?

Dangerous Interactions with Pharmaceutical Agents: St. John's wort, goldenseal, and grapefruit

Many pharmaceuticals are metabolized by the metabolic detoxification enzymes described in chapter 2. Although these enzymes undoubtedly evolved to detoxify potentially toxic constituents in the natural food supply, these same enzymes play a very significant role in metabolizing and excreting human drugs. Either inhibition or induction of these metabolizing enzymes can change the extent of exposure to the biologically active forms of therapeutic drugs by increasing or decreasing their degradation and/or their elimination from the biological target cells or the body.

The most important of these metabolizing enzymes is the family of cytochrome P450 enzymes (CYP enzymes). A number of herbal supplements have been shown to interact with these CYP enzymes, causing either increases or decreases in their activity. This is an important health issue because it is estimated that 20-30% of prescription drug users take herbal dietary supplements concurrently with their medications, often without notifying their physicians (see, *e.g.*, Gurley *et al.*, 2008). Furthermore, 70% of regular users of botanical supplements also take prescription medications (Gurley *et al.*, 2012). There are many molecular variants of these CYP enzymes, and each has specificity for a different set of chemicals. Among the most important in regard to their effects on prescription medications are CYP3A4, which metabolizes almost 50% of all prescription medications, and CYP2D6, which is estimated to metabolize approximately 30% of all medications. Some individuals carry mutations that affect the activity of these enzymes, increasing their sensitivity to inhibitory effects on these enzymes. This further complicates a situation that is already extremely complex due to the extensive number of chemical constituents in herbal products that could potentially affect these enzymes (Gurley *et al.*, 2012).

A classic example of a commonly used herbal product that has been shown to interact dangerously with therapeutic medications is St. John's wort. St. John's wort is an herb commonly marketed to relieve or prevent depression. Although a claim that it "relieved, or prevented, depression" would technically classify the product as a drug, and therefore make it subject to the rigorous safety and efficacy testing requirements of pharmaceuticals, the testing requirements are avoided by instead making general health claims allowed under DSHEA. Common claims are that it "supports mood", "promotes mental health and/or well-being", "supports emotional balance", is an "aid to healthy sleep", or promotes "positive mood". It is one of many herbal products sold with the intent to be used as a drug but exempted from safety and efficacy testing by claiming that it is a natural herb with a general health benefit. Although there is evidence that it may actually be beneficial in regard to improving mood, it has been shown to cause interactions with some drugs that lead to loss of drug effectiveness with serious consequences. This was first recognized in 1999-2000 when several reports appeared linking St. John's wort use to drastic reductions in blood concentrations of the immunosuppressant drug cyclosporine, thereby causing rejection of grafts in transplant patients. This led to further studies that subsequently showed clinically significant effects on a variety of different drug classes, including other agents that suppress the immune system, anticoagulants, anticonvulsants, antifungals, cancer chemotherapeutics, hormonal contraceptives, and others. These effects are generally due to activation of receptors that increase the activity of CYP3A and CYP2C metabolic enzymes and also increase cellular transporter activity that removes drugs from cells. Because of the broad range of susceptibility of many drugs to St. John's wort-mediated interactions, St. John's wort has been banned in France and several other countries.

In contrast to St. John's wort, which in most cases decreases drug exposure by enhancing metabolism and transport out of cells, goldenseal, a product widely sold for the prevention of colds and respiratory tract infections, is a potent inhibitor of CYP2D6 and CYP3A4 and increases exposures to drugs metabolized by these enzymes.

Such interactions are not limited to herbal supplements, but can also occur from common foods. One example is grapefruit, which has been shown to be a very potent inhibitor of CYP3A4. Consumption of grapefruit or grapefruit juice with certain blood-pressure lowering drugs, or cyclosporine for prevention of rejection of organ transplants, can cause elevated levels of those drugs in the blood, thereby making side effects more likely. Another example is chocolate, which can interact with monoamine oxidase inhibitors that are used to treat depression, leading to increased drug exposure and a sharp rise in blood pressure. Many other interactions are known and certainly even more remain unknown.

Interactions with prescription medications are considered such an important problem that the FDA maintains a website (www.fda.gov/ForConsumers/ConsumerUpdates/ucm096386. htm) that provides information about potential interactions between dietary supplements, foods, and various drugs. This site also includes a provision for consumers to sign up to receive e-mail updates about potential harmful interactions. Such information is also frequently included in the drug information sheets that come with prescription medications, and both pharmacists and consumers should review and heed those warnings to avoid unanticipated adverse effects.

Acute Liver Toxicity from Herbal Supplements: A recognized problem with as-yet unidentified specific causes

Acute liver failure, sometimes requiring liver transplantation, has been repeatedly reported in young otherwise healthy individuals, often bodybuilders using combination herbal products to augment bodybuilding practices or to promote slimming due to "fat burning" properties (*e.g.*, Navarro *et al.*, 2014, 2016; Krishna *et al.*, 2011). One major study, conducted by physicians involved with U.S. referral centers that are part of the Drug Induced Liver Injury Network (DILIN), examined the causes of acute liver injury in 839 patients with liver injury that were referred to the collaborating centers during the period 2004-2014 (Navarro *et al.*, 2014). The DILIN was established in 2003 to identify, enroll, and characterize cases of liver injury attributable to medications and herbal dietary supplements. This network has reported herbal dietary supplements to be the second most common cause of liver injury. All 839 patients in this study were judged to have hepatotoxicity due to exposure to conventional medications, herbal products, or dietary supplements. Of these, 130 patients, or 15.5% of those enrolled in the study, were judged to have liver injury caused by herbal dietary supplements. The cases involving herbal supplements used for bodybuilding occurred mainly in young men and caused prolonged jaundice but did not result in any fatalities or liver transplants. The remaining cases involving herbal dietary supplements occurred predominantly in middle-aged women and more often led to death or liver transplantation compared to injury from medications or from the bodybuilding supplements associated with liver toxicity in young men. All 13 patients that underwent liver transplantation or died in the non-bodybuilding group taking herbal dietary supplements were women. The proportion of patients with liver injury due to herbal dietary supplements increased significantly during the period of study, to 20% by 2014. It is likely to have increased further since that time due to the increased use of such supplements. Following this study, a group of experts considered these findings and published their conclusions (Navarro *et al.*, 2016).

Although the DILIN studies, and other studies, have established very strong correlations between the liver toxicity and the use of herbal dietary supplements, the specific factors responsible for the toxicity remain unknown in most cases. This is due in large part to the complexity of the products and concurrent exposures to other potentially causative factors. Combinations of multiple products are often used and an individual product often contains multiple ingredients and mixtures of naturally occurring chemical constituents. Further, the herbal supplements are often used in combination with drug products with which they possibly interact.

Among the cases of liver injury caused by herbal and dietary supplements in the DILIN study, the major agents implicated were anabolic steroids, green tea extract, and multi-ingredient nutritional supplements. The cases involving anabolic steroids were found primarily with herbal bodybuilding products, to which such steroids are commonly added illegally. This is an ongoing problem and the FDA has instituted a special monitoring program to screen these and other products that are commonly adulterated with drugs or illegal chemicals.

Since 2006, there have been more than 50 reports in the medical literature of apparent acute liver injury with jaundice attributed to green tea extracts (Navarro *et al.*, 2016). This was considered surprising, as green tea is widely consumed throughout the world. However, different extraction procedures, concurrent use of other products or medications, or idiosyncratic reactions that occur only under certain conditions could account for toxicity in certain individuals, or certain extraction procedures or use in combination with some as-yet unknown supplement or drug could be required for toxicity. Thus, consumption of green tea extract is correlated with acute liver injury in many of these cases but a specific causative constituent has not been identified. It remains possible that some other cause, or combination of causes, is responsible.

Another suspect causative agent in cases of liver toxicity is usnic acid, which is a documented liver toxicant. However, the lack of rigorously controlled prospective studies, the complexity of the ingredients and chemical constituents in these preparations, and the confusion caused by concurrent utilization of other products in uncontrolled studies has hindered its conclusive identification as a specific causative factor. Although one product, LipoKinetix, which contains a salt of usnic acid in addition to several other ingredients, has been removed from the market due to multiple reports of its association with liver failure, the lack of clear evidence of the specific factors responsible for liver failure in otherwise healthy young adults has allowed many products that contain usnic acid to remain on the market.

The supplement industry has claimed that the studies and conclusions reported by Navarro *et al.* (2014, 2016) are misleading because they don't separate products made by reputable companies from those that are adulterated by addition of either drugs or unapproved bioactive chemicals. However, this criticism is in essence asking the researcher to determine which specific products on the market are safe and well-controlled and which are not. As Navarro *et al.* point out, among other problems with the assurance of the safety of herbal dietary supplements, there are special and varied challenges when dealing with such supplements: *"For instance, the FDA does not require manufacturers to register their products with the agency, so it has limited information on the number, types, and ingredients of products in the marketplace. Product labels may not provide a full disclosure of the ingredients, their concentrations, purity, and source. There are also products that change in composition without appropriate notification of the FDA. When the Dietary Supplement Health and Education Act was first published in 1994, there were an estimated 4,000 supplements available in the United States. Currently, there are more than 80,000."* In addition, adulteration of such products is common and it is difficult, if not impossible, for the consumer or researcher to differentiate between safe and harmful products.

Fava Bean Toxicity: Some toxicities occur only in individuals with specific genetic characteristics

It has been known for centuries that fava beans are toxic to certain individuals and not to others, but only in modern times was it established that consumption of this bean leads to toxicity only in individuals with specific genetic mutations. These mutations cause a deficiency of a key enzyme responsible for preventing the toxic response. As is often the case in scientific investigations, an understanding of the factors that cause this toxicity was achieved only when several different lines of scientific research allowed the clues presented by the intriguing characteristics of this toxicity to be assembled into a complete picture of the responsible mechanism. It is now known that genetic defects that cause a deficiency of the enzyme glucose-6-phosphate dehydrogenase (G6PD) are required for the toxicity of the responsible constituents of fava beans to be expressed. In individuals with one of these genetic mutations, consumption of fava beans results in the destruction of red blood cells and this is the cause of fava bean toxicity. The technical name for this toxicity is hemolytic anemia (red blood cell deficiency caused by lysis of red blood cells). It has been estimated that about 400 million people carry mutations that lead to G6PD deficiency.

These mutations are found mainly in world regions where malaria occurs, or has occurred historically. It has been shown that these genetic mutations cause resistance to malaria, and it is believed that this property led to evolutionary selection for these genetic mutations in these parts of the world. One of these regions is the Mediterranean area, where fava beans are commonly consumed as a food. Thus, this is a region where fava bean toxicity has been particularly prevalent. However, it was not the study of fava bean toxicity that led to the discovery of the role of G6PD deficiency in red blood cell damage and ensuing toxic effects. Rather, a drug used to treat malaria, primaquine, exhibited the same type of toxicity caused by fava beans. Like fava bean toxicity, primaquine toxicity occurred in certain individuals but not others. This "primaquine sensitivity" was studied and shown to be linked to G6PD deficiency. Once the mechanism of primaquine toxicity was understood, it was recognized that individuals with G6PD deficiency were susceptible to hemolytic anemia caused by several different causative agents, including fava bean constituents, certain infections, and other drugs that caused hemolytic anemia. The common feature of these toxicities was the production of reactive oxygen molecules by the responsible agents. People with normal G6PD production maintained a high level of antioxidant protectants in their cells whereas those with G6PD deficiency were deficient in these antioxidant defenses and therefore developed toxicity. In the case of fava bean toxicity, divicine and isouramil, chemicals that exist in plants as sugar conjugates called vicine and convicine, are the principal components of fava beans responsible for the development of this toxicity.

G6PD deficiency is present mainly in males, because the responsible gene is found on the X chromosome and males have only a single copy of this chromosome. This allows the mutation to be fully expressed in males. Females have two copies of the X chromosome, one of which is inactivated during development. Therefore females that carry a single mutation in the G6PD gene have a mixture of cells, half of which are deficient and half of which are normal. It is very rare to have the mutation in both copies of the X chromosome, so females rarely have the same degree of deficiency as do males. If this sounds complicated to non-scientists, I apologize but point out that it is necessary to understand these basic scientific issues in order to not be misled into thinking that it is a simple matter to have confidence in the safety of products and constituents that have not been rigorously studied by knowledgeable scientists that understand the factors that may obscure causative associations between product exposures and adverse health effects.

This case is a prototypical example of the influence of genetic variation on toxicity. Others are known and doubtless there are many others waiting to be discovered. A summary of glucose-6-phosphate dehydrogenase deficiency and favism, along with relevant references, is available (Wikipedia, 2016a).

Lychee and Ackee Toxicity: Association with deaths and encephalitis in children

For years the cause of an illness that caused the deaths of hundreds of children each year in the Bihar province of India, in Vietnam, and in Bangladesh, and left many others brain-damaged, remained unknown (Pulla, 2015; Spencer and Palmer, 2017). These outbreaks of neurologic illness have been known for more than 20 years, but only recently has a series of reports shown that the most likely cause is a toxic factor in the lychee (litchi) fruit that ripens in the summer in these regions—the same time at which the outbreaks occur. Early investigations focused on the possibility that pesticide exposure or viral infection was the cause of this disease, but recent studies suggest that α-(methylene cyclopropyl)glycine (MCPG), a neurotoxic amino acid, is the most likely cause. The outbreaks in the Muzaffarpur district of the Bihar state of India coincide with the month-long lychee harvesting season. The illness typically occurs in the middle of the night and tends to occur at highest frequency in malnourished children. This is consistent with the fact that MCPG causes low blood sugar (hypoglycemia), that low levels of blood sugar are consistently found in the affected individuals, that the lowest blood sugar occurs in the middle of the night, and that malnourished children would be expected to be the most sensitive to this effect. Because the illness does not occur uniformly in all exposed children, it is likely that a combination of factors plays a role. It is suggested that nutritional status as well as variable content of the toxin, or group of toxins, in the fruit are important co-factors.

The characteristics of the lychee-associated neurotoxicity correspond closely with those of a syndrome that occurs in the West Indies and Africa and is caused by ackee, a fruit in the same family as the lychee. This syndrome is best-known in Jamaica, where ackee consumption is associated with a hypoglycemic encephalopathy that occurs mainly in malnourished children. Ackee, especially when unripe, contains the toxin hypoglycin A, an amino acid related to MCPG that also causes acute hypoglycemia. This is believed to be the basis of the West Indian illness. In Jamaica, the illness is referred to as Jamaican vomiting sickness, although vomiting may not occur in all cases.

Although it can still be argued that the causative agent in the lychee-associated syndrome has not been conclusively proven to be MCPG-induced hypoglycemia, in part because exposures to MCPG have not been carefully measured and correlated with the clinical outcome and in part because the predisposing factors that cause some but not others to develop the syndrome are incompletely understood, the overall body of evidence suggests very strongly that toxins in lychee and ackee produce a similar syndrome that includes severe hypoglycemia and often neurologic damage and death. There are some observed differences in the pattern of these related illnesses that indicate that variation in toxin content and composition, as well as predisposing factors such as nutritional status and level of glycogen/glucose stores, play a role in the onset of toxicity. Based on the current findings of the critical role of blood glucose levels, recommendations have recently been made to rapidly assess and correct hypoglycemia in these cases, and implementation of these recommendations in Muzaffarpur resulted in an almost 30% decrease in mortality.

As in other examples, even with the very strong clues provided in the above case by a very specific patient population that developed characteristic severe symptoms predominantly in a very specific time frame and in close relationship to the pattern of food use in the region, it has taken decades to substantiate the cause of these extreme cases of suffering and death. Even today, uncertainties remain as to the responsible causative and predisposing factor(s). Only with well-coordinated proactive laboratory and clinical studies that include careful characterization of the levels of exposure to potential causative agents can such toxicities be identified before extensive human injury has occurred.

Conclusions

The cases above show how even very toxic dietary constituents that are used for extended periods under conditions that cause severe harm can remain undetected unless carefully controlled scientific investigations are undertaken to identify the harmful effect, or unless chance events bring the problem to light. The *Aristolochia* story, like the example of cigarette smoking and lung cancer discussed in the next chapter, illustrates how difficult it can be to establish causality even in the case of severe life-threatening or lethal toxicities. This case illustrates that even many years of focused research can be insufficient despite strong clues that suggest that a severe effect is due to an unusual exposure in a specific subgroup of individuals. In this case the chance occurrence of a second poisoning episode finally drew attention to the causative factor. The ephedra case is an example of a traditional Chinese medicine that was used for thousands of years before adverse effects and deaths due to its use were recognized. Even though its use was banned in the United States much controversy and the presentation of supposed proof of safety by the companies that marketed it delayed its removal from the marketplace. The Fen-Phen case demonstrates that even when a specific adverse event reporting system is in place, as is the case with prescription drug products, an extremely serious toxicity may go unrecognized. The St. John's wort and grapefruit examples show that product uses that would normally be safe are sometimes toxic in combination with exposure to another substance. In these cases, a dietary supplement and a common food, respectively, modify the metabolism of prescription drugs and thereby cause them to be either toxic or ineffective at doses that would normally be safe. Finally, the fava bean story is a case in which genetic differences among individuals determine whether a particular food is safe or toxic.

Even when a specific toxic syndrome is recognized, years of research may be required to identify the causative agent. The examples presented illustrate that severe or fatal human poisoning may occur from commonly occurring plants thought to be harmless. These examples, and other cases not discussed above (such as the well-known cases of birth defects caused by the drug thalidomide and the cervical and vaginal cancers and fertility and pregnancy disorders in the daughters of women treated with diethylstilbestrol) show clearly that unexpected tragedies can be prevented only by comprehensive <u>prospective</u> safety testing of new products before they are released into the marketplace. Only prospective studies designed to identify potential toxicities, in combination with scientific assessment of the risks associated with the degree of exposure that occurs with actual product use, are able to provide assurance of product safety and to prevent tragic incidents of product-induced toxicities. In the absence of such systematic safety testing it is clearly inappropriate to conclude that a product is safe just because there is a long history of use in the absence of recognized adverse effects. Unfortunately, our current legal and regulatory system still suffers from the mistake of assuming that certain widely used products are safe to sell and use without such testing simply because they are of natural origin and have a long history of use.

Chapter 4

The Regulatory Framework:
Unequal Protection Under the Law

Perhaps the most important factor essential for assurance of product safety is the extent and quality of scientific information that has been obtained in an objective and scientifically controlled manner. It is very expensive to conduct the scientific testing necessary to evaluate the wide range of possible adverse health effects that could occur, and therefore extensive safety testing is generally undertaken only when mandated by law. Another important component of safety evaluation is control of the manufacturing process and establishment of product identity and purity standards that guarantee that safe and hygienic products are produced without the presence of contaminants, toxic byproducts of the manufacturing or handling and storage processes, or adulterants added to the product. In the absence of legal mandates to ensure that safety testing, manufacturing standards, and product identity and purity standards are implemented and verified by quality control testing, profit motives frequently override the maintenance of these rigorous and expensive controls.

Unfortunately, the legal requirements for such testing and product quality standards vary dramatically across different types of products. In addition, the burden of proof for establishing safety or proving harm varies with the type of product. For some the product sponsor must establish safety to the satisfaction of a regulatory agency prior to selling the product, whereas for others the product may be sold with minimal or no safety testing and the regulatory agency must demonstrate harm or unacceptable risk of harm before regulatory action can be taken.

A Brief History of Food, Drug, and Pesticide Safety Laws

The history of product safety legislation shows that regulations requiring scientific studies of product safety and maintenance of rigorous manufacturing controls have generally been enacted only following either a tragic poisoning incident or a written exposé that created public outrage and moved lawmakers to enact such controls. The history of the legislative requirements for safety testing of foods, food ingredients, pharmaceuticals, and pesticides has in each case followed this pattern. This and subsequent chapters provide a brief synopsis of the requirements for some important classes of products and include a summary of the types of testing that are required for major product groups. I focus here on the major federal laws that apply to foods, food additives, drugs, dietary supplements, cosmetics, and pesticides sold in interstate commerce in the United States, although states also have laws that apply to products used or sold within that state. I also touch on organic food products, a category that I believe is poorly understood by most consumers, and also on genetically modified or bioengineered foods and food crops.

A national food and drug law was proposed as early as 1880 by Peter Collier, Chief Chemist of the U.S. Department of Agriculture, which then had regulatory authority over foods and drugs. His successor, Harvey Wiley, then championed this first food and drug law but it was not until the book *The Jungle* by

Upton Sinclair in 1906 graphically described the unhygienic and uncontrolled food processing practices at the Chicago stockyards that public outrage finally provided the impetus to enact laws that controlled these activities. The first comprehensive law, The Pure Food and Drug Act, was passed in 1906. This landmark law was the precursor to our current food, drug, and cosmetics regulations. In addition, the Federal Meat Inspection Act was passed on the same day.

The first major expansion of the 1906 Act came in 1938, following a tragic incident in 1937 in which more than 100 deaths were caused by a toxic solvent, diethylene glycol, used in the pharmaceutical preparation "elixir sulfanilamide". At the time, there was no requirement for testing of pharmaceuticals for either safety or effectiveness prior to selling them. Under the laws in place in 1937, the only penalty awarded following litigation against the company marketing the lethal drug product was a fine levied for mislabeling the drug as an "elixir" because it did not contain alcohol (an "elixir" was defined as a drug dissolved in alcohol). This incident resulted in the passage of legislation that had been under discussion but had stalled because of the lack of sufficient support necessary for passage. The resultant legislation—the 1938 Food, Drug, and Cosmetic Act—instituted comprehensive requirements for safety testing of drugs and laid the foundation of current safety standards for foods, drugs, and cosmetics. Nonetheless, as described below, many gaps in safety assurance remained—and some remain to this day.

Another tragic incident, the occurrence of birth defects among more than 10,000 children born to women in 40 countries treated with the sedative and anti-emetic drug thalidomide during the 1950s, refocused attention on the need to fill some of these gaps and helped build support for passage of the Kefauver-Harris Amendments to the Food, Drug, and Cosmetic Act in 1962. Among other provisions of these amendments, it was required for the first time that a drug must be demonstrated to be effective for its intended therapeutic use before it could be sold in interstate commerce. In other words, prior to this amendment a drug could be sold without demonstrating that it actually provided a health benefit. This incident also resulted in greater emphasis on premarketing testing for adverse reproductive effects. Before this time, testing for the ability of drugs to induce birth defects was not a required part of the testing performed to assess the safety of drugs.

Analogous to the catalysis of the passage of the first comprehensive food and drug laws by the publication of *The Jungle*, publication of the book *Silent Spring* by Rachel Carson in 1962 is credited with catalyzing the environmental movement that led to a ban on the use of the pesticide DDT, to the creation of the U.S. Environmental Protection Agency, and to passage of the Federal Insecticide, Fungicide, and Rodenticide Act (FIFRA) that regulates the safety evaluation and use of pesticide products. FIFRA and its associated regulations mandate an extensive series of safety studies similar to the nonclinical testing requirements for pharmaceuticals and food additives, in which potential adverse human health effects are rigorously evaluated in laboratory studies. Similar to the requirements for the testing of pharmaceuticals, studies that define the absorption, distribution, and metabolism of the agent and of its potential health effects are required. The health effects studies include studies of both short- and long-term effects, including the potential to induce cancer and reproductive, developmental, and neurological effects. In addition, studies to evaluate effects on the environment and wildlife are also required prior to approval for marketing. Major impurities in the product and their potential effects must be evaluated and the method of synthesizing the product, along with standards for its identity and purity, must be established, reviewed, and approved. Based on the extensive data from the required studies, a careful analysis of potential risks at various exposure levels must be conducted and safe residue levels established before pesticides can be used on a food crop. After approval for sale, the government conducts periodic market basket surveys to verify that the established safe residue levels are not being exceeded.

General Structure of Safety Laws and Regulations

Because the regulatory framework that applies to each product class is a major determinant of the extent of available scientific information that can be used to evaluate the risk of adverse health effects, it is important to have an understanding of the differences among the requirements for the safety evaluation of various products. In particular, it is critical to understand two key features of the laws and regulations that apply to different product classes: 1) whether or not the products are required to undergo rigorous safety testing by the manufacturer or seller of the product (referred to in many regulations as the product Sponsor) and whether the results of those studies must be reviewed and approved by a government regulatory agency before the product can be sold, or 2) whether the product can be sold without testing and the responsible regulatory agency is restricted from taking regulatory action unless it demonstrates actual harm or unacceptable risk of harm. In other words, for some products the government regulatory agency has the burden of proof to demonstrate harm or unreasonable risk of harm before taking regulatory action whereas for others the manufacturer or seller has the burden of proof to demonstrate safety to the regulatory agency before the product can be sold. This is such an important distinction that a subsequent chapter is devoted to a more detailed discussion of the impact on product safety of the legal burden of proof and whether it rests on the product sponsor or on the government regulatory agency.

For most people, foods and drugs constitute the major sources of their daily intake of foreign chemicals (chemicals not produced by our own bodies). For many people, ingestion of botanical supplements is another major source of such exposure.

Although environmental exposures often receive more attention, and can be significant sources of exposure to toxic agents in certain circumstances, chemical exposures *via* foods, drugs, and dietary supplements are usually significantly greater. Although the laws regulating the sales of food additives, drugs, and pesticides have stringent requirements for safety determination and for maintenance of chemical identity and purity, it may be surprising that foods are much more loosely regulated and that the prevailing laws assume that common foods are inherently safe as long as they have a history of use. However, foods contain complex mixtures of natural chemicals, including those produced by the food plants for defense against predators, and so the assumption that they are inherently safe may not be entirely accurate.

For each class of chemicals to which we are exposed, there are specific requirements for product testing that are determined by a hierarchical set of laws, regulations, and guidelines. The governing laws are the Federal Food, Drug, and Cosmetic Act (FFDCA) in the case of foods, drugs, and cosmetics, the Federal Insecticide, Fungicide, and Rodenticide Act (FIFRA) in the case of pesticides and pesticide residues, and the Dietary Supplement Health and Education Act (DSHEA) in the case of dietary supplements. These laws set forth the legal requirements but do not specify in detail how testing is to be conducted. They do, however, empower the responsible federal agency, or agencies, to administer the law, to issue rules and regulations, and to specify in more detail the requirements that must be met. Rules and regulations are issued by the Federal Agencies that are responsible for administering the law, and these are more detailed requirements that are enforceable under the laws. These rules and regulations are codified in *The Code of Federal Regulations* (CFR), published by the Office of the Federal Register. The CFR is publicly available and is divided into 50 titles that represent broad areas subject to federal regulation. Title 21 deals with foods and drugs and is available at https://www.ecfr.gov/cgi-bin/text-idx?SID=3ee286332416f26

a91d9e6d786a604ab&mc=true&tpl=/ecfrbrowse/ Title21/21tab_02.tpl. These regulations must be followed and are much more detailed than the laws, which set forth requirements only in general terms. Even more detailed than these regulations, specific details of expected safety and efficacy testing are set forth in "guidelines" or "guidances" (different agencies and international organizations use different terminology for these) published by the responsible federal agencies or by international agencies or organizations that are recognized by U.S. federal agencies. These guidelines set forth detailed expectations of how testing is conducted and interpreted and how manufacturing, product identity, and purity standards are implemented and verified. These guidances and guidelines are technically not legally binding, but because they set forth the detailed expectations of the responsible agencies they are generally followed closely by product sponsors required to perform testing unless there is a clear and overwhelming scientific justification for an alternate approach. In the case of pharmaceuticals, for example, these include a large number of guidances issued by the FDA, guidelines issued by the Organization for Economic Cooperation and Development (OECD), and guidelines issued by the International Conferences on Harmonisation of Technical Requirements for Registration of Pharmaceuticals for Human Use (ICH). The U.S. has agreed, under treaty, to accept testing guidelines issued by the OECD, and the FDA and the pharmaceutical regulatory agencies in Europe and Japan have agreed to adopt guidelines approved *via* the ICH process. Thus, in the case of pharmaceutical testing, there is a highly detailed set of rules and guidelines for comprehensive safety and efficacy testing, developed by regulatory scientists within the FDA, consulting scientists outside the Agency, and working groups comprised of expert international scientists, that are followed to ensure comprehensive and consistent testing and interpretation, manufacturing and product identity standards, and purity assurance.

This testing must be conducted and submitted to the FDA for evaluation prior to selling the product.

Similar processes, but involving in some cases different international scientific and regulatory organizations, are in place for the evaluation of new food additives and pesticide residues. Intentional food additives that are introduced after January 1958 are regulated by the FDA under the Food, Drug, and Cosmetic Act and must meet similar requirements to those described above for pharmaceutical products and commercial pesticides. Comprehensive testing for possible adverse health effects as well as documentation of the need for and effectiveness of the additive for its proposed purpose are required, as are establishment of identity, purity, and stability standards. Nonetheless, many consumers go to extreme limits to avoid even small amounts of food additives, believing that all commercial food additives are deleterious and should be avoided. This is particularly ironic in view of the fact that consumers are often willing to pay far greater prices for "additive free" food products but then seek out "natural" products that contain greater quantities of similar types of chemicals that have not been tested for safety at all. An example of the illogical behaviors of this type is the consumer who will avoid foods that contain tiny amounts of antioxidant food additives such as BHA or BHT (maximum permitted total BHA plus BHT is 0.02% or less depending on type of food; U.S. Code of Federal Regulations 2017), chemicals that have been studied extensively and shown to be extremely effective at preventing harmful auto-oxidation of foods at low levels and proven by extensive research to be without adverse biological effects at exposure levels relevant to their concentrations in food—and then will move to the next aisle of the supermarket to purchase a product such as açaí berries, which contain much greater levels (0.25-0.35% in commercial berries) of chemically similar antioxidants that have not been subjected to the same rigorous biological studies and may contain other unknown and untested substances (Pacheco-Palencia *et al.*, 2009). This type of choice is driven by the same situation discussed above in the case of pharmaceutical products, namely that those products that require careful extensive safety testing and careful documentation of all observed toxic effects at exaggerated doses are often maligned by marketers of products that do not require testing. These vendors often cite out-of-context irrelevant health effects that have occurred at grossly exaggerated exposures not relevant to the actual product use and claim that the "natural" product lacks these effects when in fact the natural product has never been tested under similar conditions.

Food additives and pharmaceuticals are regulated under the Food, Drug, and Cosmetic Act, supported by regulations that require extensive safety evaluations and rigorous manufacturing controls prior to approval for sale of the product. In the case of pharmaceuticals, human clinical trials that demonstrate that the drug has the beneficial effects that are claimed and that safety has been demonstrated are required in addition to carefully designed laboratory studies. The clinical trials must be designed so that both the investigators and study subjects are unaware of the identity of the treatment, and therefore preconceived biases cannot influence the observations and conclusions. These important types of studies are referred to as "double-blind" studies, and they are essential to eliminate the potential biases of the study subjects and investigators when they are recording observations. The thorough testing required for the approval of food additives and pharmaceuticals provides assurance that the safety and health benefits (in the case of pharmaceuticals) and functional improvement of foods (in the case of food additives) claimed have been demonstrated both in humans and in laboratory studies in unbiased investigations, based on careful observation and recording of all harmful or undesirable effects at the exposure levels intended to be used as well as at exaggerated doses that are used to determine the margin of safety between the usage level and higher levels that would produce undesirable effects. All these studies must be conducted or sponsored by the company that proposes to produce and market the substance (conducted by the company or contracted to a testing company or organization), at the expense of the sponsoring company, and to the satisfaction of the FDA. In addition, after the FDA has approved the product it maintains an adverse event reporting system to which physicians and individuals are asked to report any adverse effects that occur in conjunction with the use of the product.

In marked contrast, botanical supplements, or botanical extracts or concentrates, sold with the claim that they maintain or promote health (and by implication prevent disease), are regulated under the Dietary Supplement Health and Education Act (DSHEA) which does not require specific studies of safety or efficacy prior to selling the product. Importantly, this law explicitly places the burden of proof on the "United States" to demonstrate a potential for injury before taking regulatory action against these products. In other words, a botanical supplement is assumed to be safe and can be sold to the public unless the U.S. government proves the potential for injury or harm, whereas a pharmaceutical product (*e.g.*, a prescription drug) or a food additive cannot be sold until the sponsoring company has established the safety and effectiveness of the product to the satisfaction of the FDA. As an example of the disparity between these situations, the current cost of conducting the research, safety, and effectiveness studies, and regulatory application costs necessary for the development and approval of each novel new drug product is currently estimated to exceed 2.5 billion dollars and requires numerous studies in laboratory animals, cellular systems, and in humans. There is no requirement that any research, safety, or effectiveness studies be done before marketing a botanical supplement, as long as it was marketed in the U.S. prior to 1994 and an advertising claim is not made that it is intended to treat, cure, or prevent any specific disease. In practice, the intent to prevent or treat disease is often strongly implied, or even claimed directly, in the advertising of such products.

The introductory section of the Dietary Supplement Health and Education Act makes clear that Congress has assumed, *a priori*, that it can generalize about the safety and effectiveness of the ingestion of botanical products without evaluating the types of rigorous scientific data that are required prior to the sale of pharmaceuticals or food additives. The introduction to this law begins by stating that Congress finds dietary supplements to be safe within a broad range of intake, and that legislation is necessary to ensure access of consumers to these products "*in order to promote wellness*".

Thus, Congress instituted this law because of the natural mistake (in my view a great mistake) of pre-supposing that these botanical products are inherently safer and more effective than conventional drugs and food additives. They are therefore widely available to consumers without the rigorous testing required of the former products. Clearly there was also a belief that these products were being overregulated by the government and that they should be free from the perceived "restriction" that demonstration of safety and efficacy in carefully designed and controlled studies is necessary prior to selling the product. This permits the marketers of these types of products to bypass the requirements for many millions of dollars of safety testing. To comply with the law they must simply place on the container a small printed notice stating that the health claims made have not been evaluated by the Food and Drug Administration and that the product is not intended to treat, cure, or prevent any disease. The FDA has not evaluated the safety of most of these types of products, nor is there a requirement that the company selling the product has even evaluated the safety in a single study—although these latter facts are not required be printed on the product label. Thus, the distinguishing feature that determines whether a product that makes a beneficial health claim is regulated under the requirements of the Food, Drug, and Cosmetic Act, which requires extensive safety and efficacy testing, or under DSHEA, which allows the product to be sold without testing, is the specific wording of the health claim made for the product rather than the way it is actually used in practice. If the product claims to cure, mitigate, or prevent a disease, it is classified as a drug and is subject to extensive laboratory and human testing. If it is claimed that the product promotes good health of people or of a particular organ or tissue, then the product is presumed to be a nutrient, to be inherently safe, is regulated under DSHEA, and can be sold without safety or efficacy testing. A new dietary supplement or ingredient in a supplement introduced into the market after 1994 requires notification of the FDA that sale of the product is intended, along with a statement of why it is believed to be safe, but no specific safety tests are mandated and marketing may be initiated without approval by the FDA.

The DSHEA law thus creates major loopholes whereby an agent actually intended to reduce the incidence of a disease, such as prostate cancer for example, can be legally sold if it is labeled "promotes good (prostate) health", even though the intent of the product is a reduced incidence of excess prostate growth and/or development of precancerous lesions and prostate cancer. If this same agent were packaged in a container that stated that it "prevented or reduced the risk of prostate cancer" or "reduced the risk of benign prostatic hyperplasia" it would be considered to be a drug and would be regulated under the stringent requirements of the Food, Drug, and Cosmetic Act. Thus, by claiming instead that it promotes prostate health it can be sold with essentially no testing as long as the statement that FDA has not evaluated the health claims is included on the package. To a scientist such as myself, it is not sensible that regulatory requirements for safety evaluation and production standards would be based on whether a package label states that the product "promotes health" or "is intended to treat, cure, mitigate, or prevent a disease" rather than on uniform requirements for adequate scientific evaluation of safety and determination of the inherent biological properties of the product. Indeed, adequate protection of public health requires the latter.

It is not my intent to argue for or against the relative safety of the general classes of substances thought of as natural *vs.* those classified as man-made or synthetic, as I do not believe that such generalizations are meaningful. Rather, I hope to show that such generalizations are counterproductive and to demonstrate that many natural and synthetically produced chemicals each have benefits but also have the potential to be toxic. The important point is that assurance of the safety of any type of product requires careful and comprehensive safety testing in conjunction with production controls that ensure a consistent and well-characterized end product. Without specific prospective safety studies, we cannot know the potential of the product to cause certain types of adverse biological effects. Without production controls and requirements for product characterization, we cannot be assured that impurities, contaminants, or variable chemical composition do not result in variable toxic properties in different product lots. Without determining the nature of any impurities, contaminants, or degradation products and conducting appropriate testing on them, we cannot know if they present a safety problem.

Pesticides, in particular, are generally perceived as highly toxic because they are designed to kill insects, microbial contaminants, or rodent pests. Because they are toxic to the target organism, it may seem logical that they must therefore present a health risk to humans. However, the Federal Insecticide, Fungicide, and Rodenticide Act and its associated regulations require that pesticides undergo extensive safety testing comparable to that required for drugs and food additives. Conservative methods are then applied to set safe exposure limits that are well below those that have been found to cause adverse effects. Additionally, there are requirements that products be analyzed to assure that legal regulatory limits of pesticide residues are not exceeded. As has been discussed, plants have evolved to produce endogenous chemicals that serve as natural pesticides and chemical deterrents to predation, but there is no regulatory requirement for systematic testing of these constituents and/or of predator-resistant plants (including those that are selected for cultivation or bred for the purpose of increased pest resistance for use by organic farmers). Thus, the toxic potential of these endogenous pesticides is generally unknown and there is no requirement to set safe levels that assure margins of safe exposure comparable to those required for synthetic pesticides. Again, the presumption that natural pesticides are necessarily safer than those synthesized by man is unsubstantiated. The current regulations in fact provide more protection to the consumer against potential effects from pesticide residues in marketed products than is the case with the naturally occurring chemical constituents of disease- and predator-resistant plant varieties that are cultivated for the organic foods marketplace.

Although it is desirable that government regulations for product safety should ensure comparable protection to consumers for all types of product use, unfortunately, the health and safety laws have never been standardized to require comparable safety testing and comparable levels of safety assurance across different types of products. In fact, the regulatory framework for assuring the safety of different products is so complex that even regulatory health scientists often do not fully appreciate the requirements of the laws and regulations that apply to products other than those under their immediate jurisdiction. Even within a single regulatory agency, such as the FDA, the requirements for specific products under their jurisdiction vary in the extreme. For example, although foods, food additives, drugs, dietary supplements, and cosmetics are all regulated by the FDA, food additives and drugs must be tested extensively and approved by the FDA before sale is permitted but conventional foods, dietary supplements, and cosmetics may be sold without premarket testing or approval (except for certain hair dyes). Also, in many cases products already on the market at the time new laws were passed are granted "grandfather status", and are thereby exempted from the requirements that apply to products in the same category that are introduced after passage of the law. For example, such "grandfathering" has been established under the food additives and dietary supplements regulations established under the Food, Drug, and Cosmetic Act Amendment of 1958 and the Dietary Supplement Health and Education Act of 1994, respectively.

Subsequent chapters provide more information about how these divergent requirements for safety studies and manufacturing and identity standards impact the relative safety of different product classes.

Chapter 5
The Natural Mistake:
Additional Issues and Examples

It should by now be evident why it is a "natural mistake" to assume that natural products are inherently safer than products that contain synthetic chemicals. Although we have all grown up using natural products as our principal source of nutrition and it may seem logical to think of them as inherently healthy and nutritious, it does not logically follow that natural foods cannot contain harmful constituents. Also, there is a general mistrust of synthetic chemicals designed and created by humans, due in part to the many health issues that have been linked to industrial chemicals and environmental contaminants. Nonetheless, not all synthetic chemicals are harmful regardless of the degree of our exposure to them.

In order to view the relative risks of chemical exposures in proper perspective, it is necessary to understand the regulatory requirements for the safety evaluation of products and the methods used to determine allowable safe limits of the chemicals they contain. The determination of safe limits of exposure to constituents in a given product requires 1) identifying potential toxicities that could occur, 2) determining the exposure levels at which the identified potential toxicities occur, and 3) establishing the margin of safety between actual exposures and exposure levels at which the potential toxicities occur. Product safety cannot be assured unless data is available to establish the types of toxicity that are possible at high exposure levels and safe levels that assure an adequate margin of safety between allowable and potentially toxic exposures.

Unfortunately, vendors of natural products frequently mislead consumers by claiming that competitors' conventional products contain "toxic" ingredients or residues because of adverse effects identified at exaggerated exposures during this process. By claiming that a product contains toxic chemicals without considering the level of exposure in the product as it is actually used, these marketers are deceiving the consumer in two highly significant ways. First, they erroneously equate a *hazard* (something that could cause an adverse effect if exposure reached a certain level) with a *risk* (the probability that an effect will occur in a given specific exposure situation). Second, they fail to mention that the regulatory safety laws do not require that the chemical constituents of the natural product be tested in the same way as those used in conventional food production. Thus, the fact that it is required to report all toxic findings from studies of food additives, pesticides, and pharmaceutical products results in dissemination of many reports of adverse findings that are not necessarily relevant to the effects expected at actual levels of usage.

It is also noteworthy that delayed adverse effects and those that may be serious but occur only infrequently tend to be overlooked when there is an immediate and obvious benefit of a product or activity. For example, even when the only benefit is a transient simple pleasure such as that derived from cigarette smoking, users find many ways to overlook the less obvious and delayed adverse consequences—even when those consequences include a markedly elevated chance of a slow and painful death associated with lung cancer. This trait leads us to accept products that are beneficial but that may in fact have other unanticipated adverse health consequences. The greater the obvious health benefit of a particular product or substance, the more likely are we (both the general public and also scientists and regulators) to accept it as beneficial and to dismiss the possibility that it may also have other characteristics that cause less obvious or delayed adverse effects.

These issues and consumer perceptions are not unique to the United States. A well-known example in Japan was the public furor over the use of the food additive AF-2 when it was discovered to have mutagenic and carcinogenic (cancer-causing) properties. The famous Japanese scientist Dr. Takashi Sugimura, the former head of the Japanese National Cancer Center, has pointed out the dichotomy of the attitudes of the Japanese public to the cancer risks associated with the food additive AF-2 and the dietary product bracken fern shoots (fiddleheads). The use of the AF-2 food additive was opposed vehemently when it was shown to have cancer-causing properties, but consumers happily continued to eat bracken fern shoots (fiddleheads) as a dietary delicacy even though research had shown that the cancer risk from bracken consumption was approximately the same as the relative risk from the food preservative AF-2 (Sugimura, 1982). Public outcries were raised over the use of the food additive AF-2 and its use was ultimately banned, but fiddleheads continued to be sold and consumed without substantial public concern. Undoubtedly many of the same people who protested against the use of AF-2 returned home from the protests to consume bracken fiddleheads as part of their evening meal! Dr. Sugimura is well-known for his studies of the role of chemicals in our normal diets in modifying human cancer rates, and his work along with that of other cancer researchers has shown that our normal diets contain many natural and processing-induced cancer-causing (and also cancer-protective) substances. Studies of human cancer rates suggest that perhaps 32-35% of human cancers could be prevented by modifying our diets (Sugimura, 1982; Willet, 1995). Although considerable research has sought to identify the major causative and protective agents in food products and the diet, the regulatory structure and regulatory resources throughout the world remain focused primarily on chemicals used in food production and preservation and not on the chemicals that occur naturally or that form during food processing.

When assessing the risk of adverse health effects from product exposures, it is also important to recognize the difficulty of identifying specific causes of adverse health outcomes in the general population. It is particularly problematic to establish causality when an adverse event already occurs at a significant incidence and the effect does not become manifest until a substantial period following exposure. For example, if a common cancer that requires years to develop is already present at a relatively high incidence, it is very difficult to associate an exposure that occurred many years earlier with the occurrence of new cases. Not only does the occurrence of new cases not raise suspicions that a chemical exposure was the cause because the disease is considered to be common and spontaneous, but the intervening period of time between past exposures and the appearance of the disease makes it very difficult to determine which of many potential causes may be responsible. Types of disease for which these considerations are particularly problematic include cancers, birth and reproductive effects, neurological disorders, cardiovascular diseases, metabolic disorders, and others.

Although examples of serious toxicities of natural products and herbal supplements that remained undiscovered for extended periods have been discussed, it seems important to add another case that is probably the best illustration of the difficulty of conclusively linking these types of adverse health effects to toxic exposures—the association between cigarette smoking and lung cancer. According to the U.S. Centers for Disease Control and Prevention, smoking causes 80% to 90% of lung cancer deaths in the United States, and people who smoke are 15-30 times more likely to get or die of lung cancer than those who do not smoke (www.cdc.gov/cancer/lung/basic_info/risk_factors.htm). Smoking causes approximately 443,000 deaths per year in the U.S. and approximately 6 million deaths/year worldwide, including ~600,000 from secondhand smoke. It is the leading cause of cancer-related deaths in both men and women in the United States. With such overwhelming statistics, it seems that the association between smoking and lung cancer would be obvious. Nonetheless, it took more than 60 years to identify and achieve scientific consensus that cigarette smoking was the cause of a cancer that rose from a relatively low incidence to become *the leading cause* of cancer deaths in both men and women.

The widespread adoption of tobacco smoking, in particular cigarette smoking, was responsible for increasing the frequency of human lung cancers from roughly about 1% of all cancers in the late 1880s to its present position as the leading cause of cancer deaths in the U.S. In spite of the dramatic increases in lung cancer rates in Europe and the U.S. in the early 1900s and continuing until recent times, cigarette smoking was only firmly established as the principal causative agent in the last half of the twentieth century. How, once such a dramatic increase in this fatal disease was noticed, could it require a period of more than 50 years for physicians and health scientists to identify the causative factor and to reach agreement that it was indeed the principal cause of this disease?

The early history that led to the conclusion that smoking was the principal cause of the rapidly rising incidence of lung cancer has been documented by Witschi (2001). The rising rate of lung cancers was apparently first noticed in Germany. In 1878 malignant lung cancers represented only 1% of all cancers at autopsy in the Institute of Pathology at the Dresden University of Technology in Germany. In 1900 vital statistics showed a significant increase in this rate and by 1918 this percentage had risen to almost 10%. By 1927 it was more than 14%. Interestingly, the 1930 edition of the *Springer Handbook of Special Pathology* noted this dramatic increase in malignant lung tumors, but the possible causes proposed at this time did not emphasize smoking. Rather, increased air pollution caused by industry, the use of asphalt on roads, increased automobile traffic, exposure to gas in World War I, the influenza pandemic of 1918, or exposure to benzene or gasoline were considered the more likely causes. Smoking was mentioned briefly as a possible cause, but was given less weight than other factors. It is not uncommon that environmental exposures are the first suspects when an increase in the rate of a particular disease is discovered, and you will note this trend in other examples such as the *Aristolochia* story presented in chapter 3.

From 1929 to 1940, attention began to focus on smoking and a number of important publications appeared suggesting that this was the most likely cause of the increase in lung cancers. During and after this period additional studies of the correlation between smoking and lung cancer in humans and laboratory studies of carcinogenic chemicals identified in cigarette smoke and tar resulted in stronger and stronger evidence that smoking was a principal, if not *the* principal, cause of lung cancer in humans. Yet it was not until mid-1956 that the U.S. Public Health Service officially undertook an appraisal of the data relating cigarette smoking to health and not until 1964 that the first U.S. Surgeon General's report on Smoking and Health was published (CDC, 2006), reaching the firm conclusion that *"Cigarette smoking is causally related to lung cancer in men; the magnitude of the effect of cigarette smoking far outweighs all other factors."* This report also noted *"The data for women, though less extensive, point in the same direction."* However, even at this point, not all physicians and scientists were convinced. At the time of my own scientific training in graduate school, I clearly remember one of my lectures on the topic of epidemiological studies that emphasized the difficulty of establishing causal relationships—and the prime example cited was that of the linkage between cigarette smoking and lung cancer. The professor concluded that the epidemiology studies of smoking-related cancers had not established a conclusive causal relationship even when the then-current laboratory studies of the harmful effects of smoking were taken into account. The final factor that convinced even those most skeptical was the dramatic increase in lung cancer among women, which began in 1960 and increased until 1987 to the point that lung cancer surpassed breast cancer as the leading cause of cancer deaths in women. The time course of this increase correlated perfectly with the increasing prevalence of smoking among women 20-30 years earlier and resulted in a 600% increase in women's death rates from lung cancer between 1950 and 2001. Now, based on many additional laboratory and epidemiology studies, the causal relationship between smoking and lung cancer is universally accepted by the medical and scientific communities. Approximately 90% of male lung cancers and 80-90% of female lung cancers are attributed to smoking.

This case illustrates how difficult it is to establish causality even when almost the entire incidence of a fatal disease is caused by a single factor and even when the observed rate of a delayed disease increases from a very small to a very large incidence. When the background incidence of particular disease is relatively high, it is much less likely that an increase will be noticed because it is generally assumed that a highly prevalent disease is "spontaneous" and physicians expect to see many cases with little reason to suspect causation by a chemical agent. In the case of smoking and lung cancer, both cigarette smoking and lung cancer were not common before 1900 and so the association between the two should have been expected to be relatively easy to identify.

Another factor that leads people to overlook causes of low-incidence diseases is that people don't tend to think in statistical terms. For example, even though there is a very strong association between smoking and lung cancer, every family seems to have an "Uncle Harry" who smoked heavily but lived to age 93 and didn't develop lung cancer. Also, some families have an "Aunt Emily" who never smoked but still developed and died of lung cancer. This often leads people, including physicians and research scientists, to dismiss the possibility of a causative link without considering the statistical chances that lead to such occurrences. Thus, even tightly linked causative associations may not be noticed for considerable periods. Most often, such causative associations come to attention in one of two ways: 1) someone notices the strong association between the exposure and the disease outcome in humans, and this leads to specific studies designed to prove or disprove that the exposure in fact causes the disease; or 2) a laboratory study demonstrates that the exposure in question can produce the disease (for example in laboratory animals) or a biochemical change known to lead to the disease (perhaps in a cellular culture in the laboratory) and this leads to further studies that prove or disprove causation in the human population.

Establishing causation of a particular disease generally requires both epidemiology studies in humans that examine the correlation between various factors and disease incidence and also laboratory studies that demonstrate that the chemical in question does in fact have the ability to cause the specific pathological changes that occur in the disease state. Both types of studies are costly and time-consuming, and both are usually necessary before the scientific evidence is sufficient to establish causality.

The example of smoking and lung cancer illustrates the difficulty of scientifically establishing the causes of delayed adverse effects, even in the relatively straightforward case of a single factor that causes a dramatic effect. There is a marked tendency for individuals (including scientists) to overweight immediate effects and to underweight delayed effects—especially when there is a degree of uncertainty (chance) associated with the delayed effect. It is critical to understand that *the absence of evidence for a human effect is very different from evidence for an absence of a human effect.* Only when specific scientific studies designed to detect specific types of adverse effects have been conducted can it be concluded that these types of toxicity do not occur and that the product is safe under the conditions of use.

It must be kept in mind that safety evaluation is complex, and requires different types of studies to establish the causes of existing adverse health effects and to provide prospective assurance that a particular specific exposure to a new product or environmental agent will not cause harm. Epidemiology studies that search for causative associations between existing diseases and chemical, environmental, and dietary factors, for example, are not an effective means of protecting us against diseases that occur long after exposure, such as cancer, because such studies can only be conducted after the disease has occurred. In the case of cigarette smoking and lung cancer, for example, it has been found that lung cancer does not reach a high incidence until 20 years or more after initiation of smoking, and so this type of study could not identify the causative factor until a very large number of lung cancer deaths had already occurred. Thus, such studies are not useful for protecting against possible delayed health effects of a new product about to be introduced into use, because extensive harm would necessarily have occurred before effects such as cancer induction, neurological disease, or other delayed diseases could be detected.

Thus, safety assurance must be based on both systematic prospective scientific studies conducted prior to extensive exposure to new products or environmental factors and on retrospective evaluation of epidemiological findings of associations between disease outcomes and potential causative factors. In subsequent chapters we will examine in more detail the laws and regulatory practices that determine the extent of such testing for different classes of products, including natural dietary supplements, organic foods, conventional foods, food additives, pharmaceutical products, and pesticides.

Chapter 6
Herbal Supplements and "Nutraceuticals": A Lesson Learned and Forgotten

Public health tragedies and/or publications exposing unsafe practices that led to the implementation of critical safety laws and regulatory controls include the elixir sulfanilamide and thalidomide tragedies that led to the 1938 Food, Drug, and Cosmetic Act and the Kefauver-Harris Amendments to the food and drug laws, the publication of *The Jungle* that exposed unsanitary food practices and led to adoption of the first major food safety legislation, and the publication of *Silent Spring* that provided impetus for controls over pesticides. Unfortunately, the lessons learned from these previous incidents—that sensible regulation and prospective premarket testing is necessary to avoid tragic unexpected health and environmental tragedies— were apparently forgotten by those who enacted the Dietary Supplement Health and Education Act of 1994 (DSHEA).

This law allows botanical supplements, including those marketed under health claims that imply that they may prevent or ameliorate diseases, to be sold without the review or approval of any regulatory agency as long as they were sold in the U.S. prior to enactment of the law. This legislation designates the FDA as the responsible regulatory agency for dietary supplements but allows older supplements to be sold without even notifying the FDA. It also restricts the FDA from taking regulatory action against the sale of botanical supplements unless the FDA can demonstrate that the product is unsafe or that there is an unreasonable risk of harm from the product. Although it is required that the FDA be notified prior to the sale of new supplements that were not sold in the U.S. prior to the 1994 law, or supplements containing such new ingredients, specific requirements for safety testing have not been implemented and approval by the FDA is not required prior to their sale. This notification procedure does allow the FDA the opportunity to object to the sale, but the main burden to demonstrate undue safety risk is on the FDA and not the vendor or manufacturer. Additionally, such new ingredients or new supplements are often approved by the FDA principally on the basis of a long history of use as a dietary ingredient—and the examples of serious toxicities from dietary supplements presented in the previous chapters illustrate why this is an inadequate criterion of safety.

The DSHEA states that dietary supplements are, *a priori*, expected to be safe and should not be restricted from sale unless adverse health outcomes or an unreasonable risk of adverse effects have been demonstrated. Although the manufacturer or distributors of such products are in principle responsible for their safety, there is currently no law or regulation that requires a firm to disclose to the FDA or to consumers the information they have used to determine that the product is safe as long as it does not contain a new dietary ingredient. Thus many dietary supplements are marketed without FDA approval and the FDA has the burden of proof to establish that a product is unsafe in order to take regulatory action against its sale. Given the limited resources of the FDA to undertake the costly studies needed to demonstrate a lack of safety and the ease with which a manufacturer can modify the product or its composition once the FDA questions its safety, there is unacceptably wide latitude to offer for sale products for which little evidence of safety or effectiveness exists.

Under the DSHEA a dietary supplement is defined as a product taken by mouth that contains a "dietary ingredient". Dietary ingredients include vitamins, minerals, herbs or other botanicals, amino acids, and substances such as enzymes, organ tissues, glandulars, and metabolites. Dietary supplements can also include extracts or concentrates. If a product contains a "new dietary ingredient" the FDA must be notified of the intent to sell the product at least 75 days prior to offering it for sale, but the product may still be sold at the end of that period without FDA approval unless the FDA objects. A new dietary ingredient is defined as a dietary ingredient that was not marketed in the U.S. before October 15, 1994 (21 U.S.C. 350b(d)), the date that the controlling legislation for dietary supplements, the Dietary Supplement Health and Education Act, was enacted. As there is no authoritative list of dietary ingredients that were marketed prior to the 1994 DSHEA legislation, the manufacturer or distributor of the product has the responsibility to determine if the product or its ingredients were marketed before this date.

The FDA has yet to finalize its guidance document that sets forth its expectations for establishment of the safety of new dietary ingredients, but the current draft of a proposed guidance document indicates that a history of use in the diet may itself be sufficient evidence of safety as long as the dietary intake has been at least as high as the proposed supplement dose. This draft guidance on new dietary ingredients thus reflects the previous FDA policy summarized by Dr. Robert Brackett, then Director of the FDA's Center for Food Safety and Applied Nutrition (CFSAN), before the Senate Committee on Government Reform in 2006—namely that there is a requirement to notify the FDA at least 75 days prior to marketing if the supplement is a new dietary ingredient, and the criterion for acceptance of evidence of safety is *"a history of use or other evidence of safety establishing that the new dietary ingredient will be expected to be safe when used as recommended."* Unless a new guidance modifies this criterion, products will continue to be approved on this basis. As has been noted, rapidly acting acute toxicities can be identified by reviewing reports of adverse outcomes associated with the usage of specific products, but delayed or low frequency events that do not uniformly affect all individuals can only be identified by prospective and carefully controlled animal and/ or human studies. Recognizing the challenges of determining what is unsafe without requiring that specific safety information be presented by manufacturers or distributors, the FDA turned to the National Academy of Sciences, asking that a committee of experts develop a proposed framework for categorizing and prioritizing dietary supplement ingredients sold in the United States. The committee was asked to provide a framework for prioritizing safety assessments of dietary supplements and for evaluating the safety of dietary supplement ingredients. This committee used their proposed framework to develop six scientific reviews or monographs as prototypes. After developing the framework and prototype monographs, the dietary supplement industry and other stakeholders were asked to review the proposal and prototype monographs and to submit comments upon which final revisions to the report could be based. The report and proposed framework were issued in 2005 (National Research Council, 2005).

This report provides background information about the DSHEA provisions and presents a proposed framework for FDA evaluation of the safety of dietary supplements. For readers interested in these details, the report is available free of charge at the website given in the reference list to this chapter (National Academy of Sciences, 2005). The report points out many of the important principles that are discussed in more detail in chapter

9 and also emphasizes the need for adequate resources at the FDA if adequate consumer protection is to be realized. Importantly, it concludes that "*the constraints imposed on FDA with regard to ensuring the absence of unreasonable risk associated with the use of dietary supplements make it difficult for the health of the American public to be adequately protected.*" This conclusion of the National Academy of Sciences (NAS) expert committee coincides with my own—namely that the constraints of the current regulatory laws, the limited resources of the FDA, and the complexity of herbal supplements are such that the consumer cannot rely on the safety of these products.

The prototype monographs produced by this committee reveal that even the strategy proposed by the NAS committee is unlikely to be successfully implemented within the current constraints of resources, legislative restraints, and product complexity. For example, the prototype monograph on saw palmetto (a supplement used to "maintain prostate health") is a four-page document that makes clear that insufficient data are available upon which a meaningful health risk assessment could be based. Although a number of human double-blind placebo-controlled clinical trials were identified, there were serious deficiencies in the interpretation of the human studies due to a lack of con-trolled identity of the test material, and insufficient animal and *in vitro* studies had been conducted to permit any conclusions about longer-term, genotoxic, reproductive, or drug-interaction effects. Clearly, no pharmaceutical product claiming a protective effect against diseases of the prostate would have been approved on the basis of information such as that provided in the NAS prototype monograph.

Contrary to the assertion of the DSHEA that dietary sup-plements are inherently safe, numerous instances of human toxicities due to botanical dietary supplements have occurred and are documented in news reports and scientific articles. These toxicities may result from the inherent properties of the herbal supplements themselves, toxic contaminants such as heavy metals or unintended toxic herbs, or intentional adulteration with biologically active chemicals or drugs. In spite of these examples of toxic episodes, public responses have not been analogous to those elicited by the elixir sulfanilamide poisonings, the adulterated food situations described in *The Jungle*, or the environmental concerns related to pesticide use described in *Silent Spring*—all of which led to the passage and implementation of major health and safety laws. This lack of public concern about botanical supplement safety is a dramatic contrast to the public furor that often arises over the publication of even indirect laboratory evidence that suggests only a remote possibility of toxic effects of pesticides, water pollutants, or food contaminants. Even when human exposures to these chemical agents may be orders of magnitude lower than those found to cause toxicity in laboratory studies, they seem to garner far more public attention and concern than do actual instances of documented human toxicities from botanical products at levels that are actually ingested.

The expanding market for botanical products known as "nutraceuticals", nutrient products or botanical supplements marketed with claims that they promote various aspects of health, is an issue of major concern because these products are allowed to be sold without the rigorous safety testing that would be required of a drug marketed for essentially the same purpose. These claims often imply clearly that their intent is the avoidance, or even cure, of disease, which in fact should make the product subject to the extensive premarket testing and FDA review requirements of drug products. This discrepancy is permitted because a product labeled "to promote health" is exempted from the rigorous requirements for safety testing that would apply if it were claimed that it prevented or reduced the risk of disease. As a scientist who has devoted his career to research on and regulation of foods and drugs, I fail to see a clear distinction between preventing disease and promoting health. Disease is defined in *Stedman's Medical Dictionary* as "1) *an interruption, cessation, or disorder of body function, system, or organ. Syn: illness, morbus, sickness., Literally, dis-ease, the opposite of ease—when something is wrong with a bodily function.*" Health and disease are often thought of as antonyms, but in fact the spectrum of physical conditions from health to disease is a broad continuum with no distinct boundary and no clear definition. Unfortunately, the lack of a clear distinction between health and disease leaves wide latitude for the marketing of "health" products that are in fact clearly intended to prevent or mitigate disease. Such products are generally labeled as promoting the health of a particular organ, which is permissible under the DSHEA as long as the package carries a disclaimer stating that the health claim has not been evaluated by the FDA. Thus, the degree of testing of products that make health claims is determined by the statements used to describe their intended health effects rather than by the actual usage. Ironically, the public perception appears to be weighted heavily toward the idea that those products labeled as improving health, especially if they are derived from a "natural" source, are inherently safer than, and potentially as effective as, conventional pharmaceutical agents that are intended to produce exactly the same health effect—even though in the latter case rigorous testing is required to prove both safety and medical effectiveness whereas in the former no testing at all is required.

Some examples of health claims that would place a product in the category of the dietary supplement *vs.* those that would place the product in the category of a pharmaceutical drug are:

- enhances sexual performance or enhances sexual health *versus* treats sexual dysfunction
- helps maintain optimum body weight *versus* prevents obesity
- and of course, helps maintain prostate health *versus* prevents or reduces the risk or effects of prostate cancer or benign prostate hyperplasia

In addition to the labeling laws that allow latitude for fuzzy and misleading claims that comply with the law by claiming health maintenance rather than disease prevention, direct violations of labeling laws by selling products that directly claim to treat, cure, diagnose, or prevent disease but have not been approved as drugs remain surprisingly common. For example, the FDA recently sent warning and advisory letters to companies that were selling more than 65 products making illegal claims that they would cure, diagnose, treat, or prevent cancer (Long, 2017). As with most warnings of this type, the agency warned that failure to cooperate could result in enforcement actions such as seizure of the products or an injunction to shut down a company. The FDA also has the option of prosecuting the offenses, which carries a penalty of up to a year in prison, five years' probation, and a fine of either $100,000 (U.S.) or twice the gain from the offense. However, only a minor fraction of such offenses is actually prosecuted in court. Many other examples of advertising that illegally claims natural cures, treatment, or prevention of diseases by "natural" products are easily found by searching the web for terms such as "natural remedies" or "natural cures". Although the laws and existing federal regulations are clear that products that claim to treat, cure, mitigate, diagnose, or prevent any disease, are classified as drugs and are required to be tested and approved by the FDA before they can be sold, many "natural remedies" and botanical supplements continue to be sold without the required testing or FDA approvals.

The use of dietary supplements and herbal remedies in the U.S. is widespread and growing (Bailey *et al.*, 2011; Navarro *et al.*, 2014). When the DSHEA was enacted in 1994, annual sales of dietary supplements in the United States were estimated to be in excess of four billion dollars per year, with approximately 600 dietary supplement manufacturers and 4000 products. These estimates are stated directly in the Act. Since that time, this market has expanded dramatically, as can be seen at a glance down the aisle of your local health food store or conventional pharmacies—which now often have entire sections of the store devoted to such products.

In a comprehensive survey reported by Bailey *et al.* (2011), approximately half of the adult U.S. population surveyed during 2003-2006 reported using dietary supplements. Multi-vitamin/multi-mineral products were the most frequently used, but botanical supplement use was also very high. Approximately 21% of women aged 31-70 and 16-18% of men in this age group reported using botanical supplements (*i.e.*, about 20% of the surveyed population). These are very high usage frequencies. The number of individuals reporting the use of supplements during the period 2003-2006 was 10% higher than in the previous survey during 1988-1994 and 17% higher than in a 1971-1974 survey. It is likely that this trend to higher levels of supplement use is continuing. Along with the increasing usage of dietary supplements, the frequency of severe toxicity associated with these products has also increased. For example, the increasing incidence of acute liver failure due to supplements use has been pointed out in both the public press and scientific literature (*e.g.*, Krishna *et al.*, 2011; *New York Times*, 2013).

Despite this widespread use of botanical supplements, and although numerous reports of serious toxicity and death from their use have appeared, there has been no public outcry for tighter safety testing requirements analogous to those that led to the enactment of new laws requiring stricter regulation, including premarket testing of the safety of drugs, food additives, and pesticides. This is not to say that concerns haven't been voiced regarding the lax regulation of the former products, but those voices have not generated a level of public concern sufficient to bring about significant changes of the lax regulatory requirements for dietary supplements.

In spite of the known cases of adverse health effects of botanical supplements and the risks of allowing the sale of untested products, including concentrates of active ingredients, botanical supplements and nutraceuticals continue to be regarded as generally safer than prescription medications used for the same ailments. It is hoped that the present discussion will focus attention on the need for modified laws and regulations and will help to move legislators and regulators toward implementation of a more uniform and effective approach to the regulation of safety across the product categories being discussed—before a widespread incident of severe toxicity occurs and provides the impetus for implementation. Since the current status of dietary supplement safety regulations seems to be similar to that of medical drugs just prior to the elixir sulfanilamide disaster, it is of interest to reflect on the following excerpt from a brief history of the elixir sulfanilamide incident, written by Carol Ballentine in 1981. This excerpt captures the poignant reaction to that tragedy and its impact on the enactment of the 1938 FDA legislation. Hopefully, a similar disaster will not be required to bring substantive change to the current dietary supplement safety regulations.

From FDA Website:
(Reproduced by permission)

FDA Consumer magazine article
June 1981 Issue

"Taste of Raspberries, Taste of Death: The 1937 Elixir Sulfanilamide Incident"

By the 1930s it was widely recognized that the Food and Drugs Act of 1906 was obsolete, but bitter disagreement arose as to what should replace it. By 1937 most of the arguments had been resolved but Congressional action was stalled. Then came a shocking development--the deaths of more than 100 people after using a drug that was clearly unsafe. The incident hastened final enactment in 1938 of the Federal Food, Drug, and Cosmetic

Act, the statute that today remains the basis for FDA regulation of these products.

"Nobody but Almighty God and I can know what I have been through these past few days. I have been familiar with death in the years since I received my M.D. from Tulane University School of Medicine with the rest of my class of 1911. Covington County has been my home. I have practiced here for years. Any doctor who has practiced more than a quarter of a century has seen his share of death.

But to realize that six human beings, all of them my patients, one of them my best friend, are dead because they took medicine that I prescribed for them innocently, and to realize that that medicine which I had used for years in such cases suddenly had become a deadly poison in its newest and most modern form, as recommended by a great and reputable pharmaceutical firm in Tennessee: well, that realization has given me such days and nights of mental and spiritual agony as I did not believe a human being could undergo and survive. I have known hours when death for me would be a welcome relief from this agony." (Letter by Dr. A.S. Calhoun, October 22, 1937)

The medicine that killed Dr. Calhoun's patients was Elixir Sulfanilamide. During September and October 1937 this drug was responsible for the deaths of more than 100 people in 15 states, as far east as Virginia and as far west as California. The drug and the deaths led to the passage of the 1938 Food, Drug, and Cosmetic Act, which increased FDA's authority to regulate drugs.

Sulfanilamide, a drug used to treat streptococcal infections, had been shown to have dramatic curative effects and had been used safely for some time in tablet and powder form. In June 1937, however, a salesman for the S.E. Massengill Co., in Bristol, Tenn., reported a demand in the southern states for the drug in liquid form. The company's chief chemist and pharmacist, Harold Cole Watkins, experimented and found that sulfanilamide would dissolve in diethylene glycol. The company control lab tested the mixture for flavor, appearance, and fragrance and found it satisfactory. Immediately, the company compounded a quantity of the elixir and sent shipments--633 of them--all over the country.

The new formulation had not been tested for toxicity. At the time the food and drugs law did not require that safety studies be done on new drugs. Selling toxic drugs was, undoubtedly, bad for business and could damage a firm's reputation, but it was not illegal.

. . .

Victims of Elixir Sulfanilamide poisoning--many of them children being treated for sore throats--were ill about 7 to 21 days. All exhibited similar symptoms, characteristic of kidney failure: stoppage of urine, severe abdominal pain, nausea, vomiting, stupor, and convulsions. They suffered intense and unrelenting pain. At the time there was no known antidote or treatment for diethylene glycol poisoning. In a letter to President Franklin D. Roosevelt, a woman described the death of her child:

"The first time I ever had occasion to call in a doctor for [Joan] and she was given Elixir of Sulfanilamide. All that is left to us is the caring for her little grave. Even the memory of her is mixed with sorrow for we can see her little body tossing to and fro and hear that little voice screaming with pain and it seems

as though it would drive me insane. … It is my plea that you will take steps to prevent such sales of drugs that will take little lives and leave such suffering behind and such a bleak outlook on the future as I have tonight."

A few simple tests on experimental animals would have demonstrated the lethal properties of the elixir. Even a review of the current existing scientific literature would have shown that other studies--such as those reported in several medical journals--had indicated that diethylene glycol was toxic and could cause kidney damage or failure. But in 1937 the law did not prohibit the sale of dangerous, untested, or poisonous drugs. Dr. Samual Evans Massengill, the firm's owner, said: "My chemists and I deeply regret the fatal results, but there was no error in the manufacture of the product. We have been supplying a legitimate professional demand and not once could have foreseen the unlooked-for results. I do not feel that there was any responsibility on our part." The firm's chemist apparently did not share this feeling; Harold Watkins committed suicide after learning of the effects of his latest concoction.

. . .

Twenty-five seizures were made under federal law. The charge was misbranding. "Elixir," FDA said, implied the product was an alcoholic solution whereas it was, in fact, a diethylene glycol solution and contained no alcohol. If the product had been called a "solution" instead of an "elixir," no charge of violating the law could have been made. FDA would have had no legal authority to ensure the recovery of the drug and many more people probably would have died.

FDA Commissioner Walter Campbell, who was then

pressing for better federal regulation of drugs, pointed out how the inadequacy of the law had contributed to the disaster. "It is unfortunate that under the terms of our present inadequate Federal law, the Food and Drug Administration is obliged to proceed against this product on a technical and trivial charge of misbranding. …[The Elixir Sulfanilamide incident] emphasizes how essential it is to public welfare that the distribution of highly potent drugs should be controlled by an adequate Federal Food and Drug law. … We should not lose sight of the fact that we had many deaths and cases of blindness resulting from the use of another new drug, dinitrophenol, which was recklessly placed upon the market some years ago. Deaths and blindness from this [drug] are continuing today. We also should remember the deaths resulting from damage to the liver that have occurred from cinchophen poisoning, a drug often recommended in such painful conditions as rheumatism. We also have unfortunate poisoning, acute and chronic, resulting from thyroid and radium preparations improperly administered to the public.

"These unfortunate occurrences may be expected to continue because new and relatively untried drug preparations are being manufactured almost daily at the whim of the individual manufacturer, and the damage to public health cannot accurately be estimated. The only remedy for such a situation is the enactment by Congress of an adequate and comprehensive national Food and Drugs Act which will require that all medicines placed upon the market shall be safe to use under the directions for use. …"

As it turned out, the Elixir experience did more than hasten enactment of the 1938 Federal Food, Drug, and Cosmetic

Act. The New Drug section, added to prevent such trage-
dies, gave the United States a new system of drug control
which provided superior protection while stimulating med-
ical research and progress. And 25 years later, it saved the
Nation from an even greater drug tragedy—a thalidomide
disaster—like that in Germany and England. Here again,
history repeated itself. A pending bill, the Drug Amendments
of 1962, was finally enacted."

Unfortunately, it appears that the above-described critical lesson learned during the period of unregulated sales and use of prescription drugs—namely that sensible regulation and prospective premarket safety testing is required if tragic health outcomes are to be avoided—has been forgotten. Let us hope that another tragedy involving botanical supplements is not required to spur reform of the current inadequate system of regulation of these products. Hopefully, action will be taken to implement more sensible regulations for botanical products and other supplements, or at least the information presented in this book will lead consumers to make more sensible choices, without the need for another incident of human suffering and death to catalyze the needed changes.

Chapter 7
Drug and Chemical Spiking of Nutraceuticals: A Particularly Serious Problem

In addition to the health risks associated with the lack of adequate safety testing and review of botanical supplement products, the laxity of the current laws and the limited resources available to the responsible regulatory agencies have resulted in inadequate control of the widespread practice of deliberately adulterating these products by adding synthetic biologically active ingredients or drugs to make them biologically active, or diluting them with inexpensive inactive ingredients to reduce the cost of production. The dangerous practice of adding illegal synthetic biologically active substances or prescription drugs to botanical supplements in order to produce a biological effect that is falsely ascribed to the "natural" product has become alarmingly widespread. This practice is termed "spiking", and is frequently practiced by unscrupulous companies or individuals.

The addition to a dietary supplement of a drug product, a chemical that has biological activity similar to a drug product, or any bioactive chemical not recognized as a nutrient or nutritional supplement is illegal. However, the complexity of the chemical composition of botanicals, the limited resources of the FDA, and the nature of the laws governing the sale and regulation of the dietary supplements make it difficult to effectively regulate these practices. Even when the regulatory agency has established that such illegal substances are present in the product prosecution is rarely pursued.

Spiking with illegal biologically active ingredients has been found with many different products but is especially prevalent among supplements promoted for sexual enhancement, weight loss, bodybuilding, and athletic performance. This makes these products particularly dangerous. The FDA is aware of this problem and has instituted a program to test these types of products in an effort to identify those that are adulterated and to remove them from the market. Unfortunately, their regulatory authority is sufficiently limited that fear of prosecution often does not deter the perpetrators. The FDA, Department of Justice, and other federal partners do in some cases pursue injunctions or seizures of products against companies that sell adulterated or otherwise illegal dietary supplements, and also bring criminal prosecutions in some cases. However, prosecutions are brought in only a minority of the cases of identified adulteration. It is clear that the surveillance programs currently in place are identifying only a fraction of the cases of actual product adulteration. The principal responses from the FDA when such spiking is brought to their attention or discovered by their limited surveillance program is to issue a warning letter to the distributor of the product asking that it be removed from the market and to provide notice of the finding to consumers and health care providers. These warning notices generally result in the voluntary withdrawal of the adulterated product by the product sponsor, but studies have shown that even when such products are removed from the market there is a very high frequency of recurrent sales of the same or a similar adulterated product.

This high rate of reintroduction of adulterated products was documented in a 2014 study by researchers from the Harvard Medical School, Cornell University, and Flora Research Laboratories. In this study researchers identified products that were found by the FDA to be adulterated and recalled from the market during the period 2009-2012 and then returned to the marketplace, supposedly now free of the illegal constituents (Cohen *et al.*, 2014). During this period 274 dietary supplements were recalled from the marketplace due to illegal adulteration with biologically active substances. The researchers identified and analyzed 27 of these products that were returned to the market and were being sold under the identical supplement name in July or August of 2013 by the same manufacturer or distributor of the product that had sold it at the time of the recall. In other words, the objective was to study the compliance with the law and to determine the degree of responsible safety management by those manufacturers and distributors of these products *after* they had previously been recalled for illegal adulteration and were then reintroduced after presumed correction of the adulteration. Of these supplements that were returned to the market and subsequently analyzed by the researchers, 66.7% contained one or more pharmaceutical adulterants! In the subset of these that were produced by manufacturers in the United States, 65% remained adulterated with banned ingredients, or approximately the same percentage as for all samples analyzed.

Among the samples analyzed, 85% of those for sports enhancement (11/13), 67% of those for weight loss (6/9), and 20% of those for sexual enhancement (1/5) were found to be adulterated during the period of 6 months to 4 years after their recall. These numbers are almost certainly underestimates of the true extent of the problem because these authors only analyzed for common adulterants that would be expected in the product type investigated. Nonetheless, these results show clearly that the practice of drug spiking is extremely widespread, even among those products that have previously been withdrawn from the market due to the FDA's identification of illegal addition of biologically active constituents. As is pointed out by the authors of this study, *"More aggressive enforcement of the law, changes to the law to increase the FDA's enforcement powers, or both will be required if sales of these* (adulterated) *products are to be prevented in the future."*

The FDA is in fact striving to improve its approaches to controlling these serious problems with adulteration, but the availability of resources continues to be inadequate given the scope of the problem. In 2006, the focus and priorities of the FDA related to the regulation of dietary supplements were summarized before the Senate Committee on Government Reform by the testimony of Bob Brackett, then Director of the FDA's Center for Food Safety and Applied Nutrition (CFSAN) (statement of Robert E. Brackett, 2006). Since this time, screening and enforcement efforts have been increased, but the testimony reveals a number of the major weaknesses of FDA's regulatory approach that have not fundamentally changed. Although the FDA is making a substantial effort to regulate botanical supplements, the difficulty of effective enforcement under the current controlling legislation makes it all but impossible to assure the safety of the multitude of such products currently being sold. As described in Dr. Brackett's testimony, during the approximately 3½ year period from October 2002 to February 2006, 588 domestic inspections were conducted and 350 warning letters of product violations were issued. Permanent injunctions were issued against five firms for distribution of dietary supplements that were deemed to be misbranded and/or adulterated with unapproved drugs, and 4000 foreign shipments of potentially unsafe or misbranded dietary supplements were refused importation. However, Dr. Brackett's 2006 summary of FDA enforcement actions included only one case of criminal prosecution related to botanical sales.

The single case of a criminal conviction cited in that testimony was not related to illegal spiking of supplements, but was a conviction related to the promotion and sale of an unapproved botanical product for the treatment of cancer. Jason Vale, President of a company marketing Laetrile, produced from apricot pits, for the treatment of cancer was first placed under injunction in 2000 by court order to prevent his company's illegal sale of this unapproved drug product for the treatment of cancer. Although studies had shown that the treatments were ineffective and the sale for cancer treatment was illegal, the court order was defied and Vale continued to sell the product under a different shell corporation. Vale was then prosecuted and found guilty of criminal contempt, and was sentenced to 63 months in prison and 3 years of supervised release. Although this was the only example presented to the Senate in 2006 as evidence of FDA's enforcement activities, FDA has recently placed more emphasis on illegal botanical adulteration and both monitoring and prosecution activities have been increased since that time.

The increased emphasis on enforcement of dietary supplement regulations is exemplified by a March 8, 2016, announcement of the U.S. Attorney General Loretta Lynch as part of 2016 consumer protection week activities. This announcement emphasized the Department of Justice's priority focus on the protection of consumers from unsafe dietary supplements. Given the wide range of responsibilities of the Department of Justice, it is significant that this was one of the priority areas selected for emphasis. This announcement notes that in the one-year period from November 2014 to November 2015 the Department of Justice had participated in greater than one hundred criminal and civil cases against dietary supplement manufacturers and marketers. Among the civil cases were those involving products making "disease claims" that would subject them to the requirements of premarketing approval as drugs and others against products that illegally contained drug products or unapproved biologically active chemicals. Fourteen of the cases were criminal prosecutions involving at least 29 individuals and entities.

A recent example (FDA, 2017) of this type of case is that of the co-owner of the Texas dietary supplement company X2 Zero Corporation, which was found to be illegally selling products adulterated with several approved and withdrawn drugs and drug analogs associated with weight loss and sexual performance, as well as violating Good Manufacturing Practices. As of 2017 this individual faces up to five years in federal prison and a possible $250,000 maximum fine for the controlled substance violation as well as one year in prison and an additional $100,000 maximum fine for violating the Food, Drug, and Cosmetic Act. Another notable case is a lawsuit brought by the state of Oregon against GNC Holdings, Inc., a major health foods and supplements store chain, for selling dietary products containing illegal and potentially dangerous ingredients, specifically BMPEA (β-methylphenylethylamine) and the unapproved drug picamilon (*Wall Street Journal*, 2015). BMPEA is a stimulant similar to amphetamine and is banned in sports by the World Anti-Doping Agency. Picamilon is used in Russia as a prescription drug to treat neurological conditions but is not an approved drug in the U.S. It is a combination of a neurotransmitter (gamma-aminobutyric acid) and niacin (vitamin B_3). The Oregon lawsuit claims that GNC staff knew of picamilon's status as an unlawful ingredient as early as 2007 but still sold thousands of units of supplements containing this ingredient up to 2015. The complaint alleges that GNC continued selling products with picamilon even after Oregon authorities contacted the company about this ingredient, and noted that it stopped selling products with BMPEA only after its suppliers received warning letters from the FDA that BMPEA is not considered a legal dietary ingredient. As of June 2017, picamilon could still be found for sale on the internet.

Despite an increased federal regulatory and enforcement focus on dietary supplement safety, criminal prosecution continues to be pursued in only a minority of the cases of identified adulteration.

A few minutes perusal of the internet shows that the marketing of supplements clearly promoted for treatment or prevention of diseases (which under the law makes them unapproved and therefore illegal drug products) remains extremely prevalent to this day. For example, an informal survey by this author of public notifications by the FDA of products adulterated by illegal spiking with prescription drugs, unapproved drug products, or other biologically active chemicals, and of notices of product recalls due to such spiking, during the period October 2015 to April 2017 (a period of approximately 1½ years) identified 208 such notices. This is certainly an underestimate of the number of FDA actions during this period, as this was not a comprehensive search but rather was just a compilation of notices that was observed by monitoring the FDA website and subscribing to one of the FDA notification services. Thus, it is clear that adulterated and misbranded botanical supplements continue to be a very significant problem and that many such products continue to be sold.

A current major focus of the FDA's efforts to identify illegal spiking is to screen those products known to have a high rate of adulteration for the most common and likely hazardous adulterants. The FDA is well aware of its limited ability to adequately regulate the safety of botanical supplements but can only optimize available resources to the extent that they are available. The following quotation from the FDA website on consumer information illustrates their concern in the case of spiking of products for sexual enhancement.

"Tainted Sexual Enhancement Products"

FDA has identified an emerging trend where over-the-counter products, frequently represented as dietary supplements, contain hidden active ingredients that could be harmful. Consumers may unknowingly take products laced with varying quantities of approved prescription drug ingredients, controlled substances, and untested and unstudied pharmaceutically active ingredients. These deceptive products can harm you! Hidden ingredients are increasingly becoming a problem in products promoted for sexual enhancement.

> **Remember, FDA cannot test all products on the market that contain potentially harmful hidden ingredients. Enforcement actions and consumer advisories for tainted products only cover a small fraction of the tainted over-the-counter products on the market.**

A similar situation exists with products for weight loss and products for bodybuilding. For example, the FDA posts a similar notice about weight loss products:

Tainted Weight Loss Products

FDA has identified an emerging trend where over-the-counter products, frequently represented as dietary supplements, contain hidden active ingredients that could be harmful. Consumers may unknowingly take products laced with varying quantities of approved prescription drug ingredients, controlled substances, and untested and unstudied pharmaceutically active ingredients. These deceptive products can harm you! Hidden ingredients are increasingly becoming a problem in products promoted for weight loss.

> **Remember, FDA cannot test all products on the market that contain potentially harmful hidden ingredients. Enforcement actions and consumer advisories for tainted products only cover a small fraction of the tainted over-the-counter products on the market.**

Although adulteration with highly biologically active chemicals is a major health and safety concern, intentional adulteration of expensive products with lower cost ingredients is also common. For example, approximately 250-300 essential oils are used in commercial fragrances, medicinal products, incenses, and other products. These products comprise a $7 billion industry, and adulteration of these expensive oils with less expensive solvents and oils is common (Schmidt and Wanner, 2016). Another example is a study of 18 samples of commercial *Ginkgo biloba*, of which at least 7 were found to be adulterated with flavonols or flavonol glycosides (Harnly *et al.*, 2012). There are many other examples of intentional and non-intentional adulteration of commercial botanical products that are far too numerous to summarize here.

Responsible botanical product companies and industry organizations are also aware of the problem with product adulteration and some have instituted their own programs to address these issues. For example, CVS Pharmacy plans to institute new standards for the dietary supplements that it sells, and intends to include a requirement for third-party testing of ingredients and of ingredients of special concern (Schultz, 2017). This program is expected to be implemented by 2019 and to cover more than 800 products and 100 supplier partners of the company. Another example is the American Botanical Council (ABC)-American Herbal Pharmacopoeia (AHP)-National Center for Natural Products Research (NCNPR) Botanical Adulterants Prevention Program, which is an international consortium of nonprofit professional organizations, analytical laboratories, research centers, industry trade associations, industry members, and other parties with interests in herbs and medicinal plants. This Program was formed to advise industry, researchers, health professionals, government agencies, the media, and the public about various issues related to adulterated botanical ingredients sold in commerce.

The Center's program is supported by more than 180 U.S. and international parties, and it publishes peer-reviewed articles on subjects related to adulteration, including reviews of specific products' adulteration and methodologies for detecting and controlling adulterants. A brief history of the initiation of this consortium and of adulteration of herbs and botanical drugs is provided by Foster (2011). Companies that sell botanical products often obtain the products from suppliers, frequently from countries outside the U.S., but the companies selling the products have legal responsibility for the safety of their products. Even though they are not required to submit safety information to the FDA prior to selling the products, they are ultimately responsible under the law for the safety of the products they sell. Thus, they are subject to regulatory enforcement for the sale of unsafe products, including prosecution for intentional illegal adulteration or suits for damages due to negligence in marketing unsafe products. Adulteration reviews by this group are helpful to responsible companies that are trying to avoid obtaining adulterated products from suppliers. They also provide background information on potential product problems to consumers. Publications by this group have included reviews of black cohosh, ginkgo, skullcap, bilberry fruit extract, pomegranate, ginseng, tea tree oil, and the substitution of synthetic antimicrobial compounds for products sold as grapefruit seed extract. Findings of adulteration, including dilution of authentic products with lower-cost ingredients and addition of specific chemicals to natural botanicals are common. This program also publishes other botanical adulterant bulletins, laboratory guidance documents, and a quarterly newsletter entitled the *Botanical Adulterants Monitor*. The program's publications are available at no cost on their website (http://cms. herbalgram.org/BAP/).

Although readers will undoubtedly be interested in the specific types of adverse effects that might occur from consumption of unsafe dietary supplements, the wide range of botanical products and possible adulterants, the chemical complexity of natural chemical constituents in these products, and the dearth of available safety studies of standardized products makes it impossible to summarize these potential effects. Only a few examples of adverse effects from some of the most commonly adulterated products can be given here. As has been noted, adulteration of weight loss products, products for enhancement of sexual performance, and products for enhancement of athletic performance and muscle building is particularly common. Examples of common adulterants in these products include sibutramine and its chemical relatives in weight loss products, tadalafil (Cialis), sildenafil (Viagra), and other phosphodiesterase-5 (PDE-5) inhibitors in products for enhancement of male sexual performance, bioactive amines in products for improved athletic performance or weight loss, and anabolic steroids in muscle-building products.

Supplements sold for male sexual enhancement are one of the most frequently adulterated products. These products very frequently contain tadalafil or sildenafil (the active ingredients in Cialis and Viagra) or chemical analogs of these or other drugs for erectile dysfunction. This is dangerous because the most frequent users of these products are elderly males who are likely to also be taking medications that lower blood pressure, such as antihypertensive drugs, nitrate drugs such as nitroglycerin, isosorbide mononitrate, or isosorbide dinitrate for angina, or alpha blockers for benign prostate disease. Interactions with these drugs can cause unsafe decreases in blood pressure or heart attack. Use in combination with excessive alcohol can also cause decreases in blood pressure. Less common, but real, risks include adverse effects on vision or on hearing.

Weight loss products are also frequently adulterated. One of the most common adulterants is sibutramine and/or its chemical relatives. Sibutramine affects the uptake of a chemical involved in neural transmission (serotonin), has anorexic (loss of appetite) properties, and causes increased blood pressure and increased heart rate. It is a risk for people with coronary artery diseases and can cause heart arrhythmias, stroke, or life-threatening interactions in combination with other drugs. It was approved in the United States for obesity treatment in 1997 but was removed from the market in the U.S. in 2010 and also withdrawn in many other countries including Canada, the European Union, Australia, the United Kingdom, India, and others. The FDA began issuing alerts about dietary supplements for weight loss illegally adulterated with sibutramine in 2009, with alerts about or recalls of 61 products in that year, but the problem continues to the present day. Other adulterants that have been found in weight loss products are:

- phenolphthalein, a laxative that was removed from the market in 1997 due to potential cancer-causing risks.

- phentermine and other bioactive amines. Phentermine is similar to amphetamine and is approved for short-term use for weight loss. It was part of the Fen-Phen combination described in chapter 3 that was withdrawn in 1997 due to heart valve damage, although this effect was attributed mainly to the fenfluramine component of the combination. Adverse effects of phentermine include elevated blood pressure, cardiac palpitation, restlessness, insomnia, nervousness, dizziness, and rare cases of pulmonary hypertension, stroke, angina, and cardiac disturbances.

- fluoxetine, a drug with biological effects similar to sibutramine, is used as an antidepressant under trade names Prozac and Sarafem. Fluoxetine affects serotonin pharmacokinetics and is associated with suicidal thinking, seizures, and heart arrhythmias in combination with certain other drugs.

- rimonabant (Acomplia, Zimulti), a weight loss drug with anorexic (appetite suppressant) properties that works by blocking cannabinoid receptors in the central nervous system. It was approved in the European Union in 2006 but was withdrawn in 2009 due to side effects including depression, severe anxiety, and suicidal tendencies. It was never approved in the United States.

- sertraline (Zoloft) is a drug approved as an antidepressant that has a pharmacological action similar to sibutramine. It is sometimes found in weight loss products. Adverse effects include diarrhea, nausea, sexual dysfunction, and a small risk of suicidal tendency in young people. It may interact with certain drugs to cause more serious effects.

- phenytoin (Dilantin) is an anti-seizure dug that causes appetite loss. Adverse effects include sleepiness, liver problems, low blood pressure, bone marrow suppression, severe skin reactions, and birth defects.

- fenfluramine, a drug that has been withdrawn due to heart valve problems and potential pulmonary hypertension.

- orlistat, an approved anti-obesity drug, the addition of which to a botanical supplement product without approval is illegal.

Muscle-building and athletic performance-enhancing products often contain androgenic steroids or non-steroidal chemicals known as selective androgen receptor modulators (SARMs), such as andarine and ostarine (Enobosarm) that are considered unapproved drugs with anabolic steroid-like effects. Use or consumption of products containing SARMs and anabolic steroid-like substances may cause acute liver injury, which is a known harmful effect of steroid-containing products. In addition, abuse of anabolic steroids may cause other serious long-term adverse health consequences including shrinkage of the testes and male infertility, masculinization of women, breast enlargement in males, short stature in children, a higher predilection to misuse other drugs and alcohol, adverse effects on blood lipid levels, and increased risk of heart attack, stroke, and death. Stimulants such as amphetamines, ephedrine, or pseudoephedrine that can cause nervousness, insomnia, elevated blood pressure, or heart palpitations, and increase the risk of cardiovascular effects such as stroke or heart attack are also found as adulterants in athletic-enhancing products. Caffeine is also often used as a stimulant to improve athletic performance and may be found as an adulterant in this class of botanical products. Methylphenidate (Ritalin), a widely used drug for attention deficit disorders is a stimulant that has been found in athletic performance and weight loss products. It can elevate blood pressure, cause anxiety, trigger circulation problems in fingers and toes, and has been associated with stroke, heart attack, and sudden death, especially in people with heart deformities or other serious heart disorders.

Consumers of botanical supplements as well as doctors and other health care providers can help the FDA identify problems with specific products by reporting adverse reactions from botanical supplements through the FDA's adverse event reporting system. Through this voluntary reporting system the FDA monitors reports of health problems associated with specific products, and when potential problems are identified they can then focus their limited resources on investigation of those high-risk products. It is a major help to the Agency in identifying potential product-related health issues and is a way to help them protect the public from serious health effects of adulterated or unsafe products. This is such an important activity that the FDA instructions for reporting such problems, found at https://www.fda.gov/food/dietary-supplements/how-report-problem-dietary-supplements are reproduced below. Readers are encouraged to use this reporting system to inform the FDA of any adverse reactions they have to botanical supplements.

How to Report a Problem with Dietary Supplements

Dietary supplements include vitamins, minerals, herbs, amino acids, whey protein, creatine, and weight loss pills. FDA does not approve dietary supplement products before they are sold to the public. Therefore, it is particularly important for consumers, health professionals, and industry members to report serious health-related reactions or illnesses (also known as adverse events) to FDA, so we can take action to protect the public from unsafe products.

Serious reactions or illnesses may include:

- *itching, rash, hives, throat/lip/tongue swelling, wheezing*
- *low blood pressure, fainting, chest pain, shortness of breath, palpitations, irregular heart beat*
- *severe, persistent nausea, vomiting, diarrhea, or abdominal pain*
- *difficulty urinating, decreased urination*
- *fatigue, appetite loss, yellowing skin/eyes, itching, dark urine*
- *severe joint/muscle pain*
- *slurred speech, one-sided weakness of face, arm, leg, vision (stroke)*
- *abnormal bleeding from nose or gums*
- *blood in urine, stool, vomit, or sputum*
- *marked mood, cognitive, or behavioral changes, thoughts of suicide*
- *visit to Emergency Room or hospitalization*

For Consumers and Health Professionals:

If you think that a dietary supplement may have caused you or someone you know to have a serious reaction or illness, immediately stop using the product and fill out a safety report through the Safety Reporting Portal (https://www.safetyreporting.hhs.gov/srp2/default.aspx?sid=495f389b-69ab-400e-a6f2-48889ea50cde) to submit your complaint to FDA.

After logging in or choosing to report as a guest, select the option "Start a new report" and choose "Dietary Supplement Report (voluntary) . . ." Please supply as much information as you can. Complete reports are the most helpful, but even pieces of information can help FDA identify potentially dangerous products.

For Industry:

Members of the dietary supplement industry may now use the reporting form on the Safety Reporting Portal (https://www. safetyreporting.hhs.gov/srp2/default.aspx?sid=495f389b-69ab-400e-a6f2-48889ea50cde) to meet the reporting requirements established in section 761 of the FD&C Act.

After logging in or choosing to report as a guest, select the option "Start a new report" and choose "Dietary Supplement Report (mandatory) . . . "

If You Need Assistance:

If you have any questions about reporting on dietary supplements, please contact DSRSupport@fda.hhs.gov. For technical support with submitting a safety report, please contact SRPSupport@fda.hhs.gov.

For information on how to report a problem with food, visit How to Report a Problem with Food (https://www.fda.gov/ Food/ ResourcesForYou/ucm334249.htm)

To encourage consumers to report cases of adverse reactions or suspicious claims in marketing, advertising, or labeling of dietary supplements or other health-related products, the FDA and the Federal Trade Commission (FTC) have recently posted a notice to consumers asking them to make such reports. This notice contains links to the FDA Safety Reporting Portal and the FTC Complaint Assistant websites. Because many consumers are not aware of which aspects of safety control, product labeling, and advertising are controlled by each Agency, this notice makes clear that the two agencies coordinate the handling of these reports and will make sure that the appropriate Agency and division receives the report regardless of which one receives it initially. Such reports are an important means by which these agencies identify problems and they also provide documentation that supports subsequent regulatory actions.

The FDA issues frequent public warnings and notices of product recalls due to illegal hidden drug ingredients. The basis of most FDA actions against such tainted products is the finding that the product contains "a hidden drug ingredient" and is therefore an unapproved prescription drug product that cannot be sold without an approved New Drug Application. The fact that the FDA chooses to apply the prescription drug law and regulations illustrates the relative strength of those regulations and the weakness of those that apply to botanical supplements. The public can subscribe to the following website "feed" to receive announcements on tainted dietary supplements. I suspect that the average reader may be surprised at the number of such reports. For the interested reader, anyone may subscribe to FDA e-mail notifications on a variety of topics, including FDA warning letters, product recalls, safety alerts, and other topics including news on diseases and conditions at https://www.fda.gov/Safety/Recalls/.

Given the unregulated nature of the botanical product market, it would be advisable for anyone inclined to take such products to monitor these notices—but a far better safety measure is to categorically avoid taking these types of products, especially those in the known higher-risk categories.

Chapter 8

Regulation of Food Products, Additives, and Pesticide Residues

This and the following chapter provide an overview of the regulatory framework, testing requirements, and enforcement authorities that apply to the different product classes under discussion. These factors determine the relative degree of safety assurance for a particular product by establishing requirements for obtaining and evaluating reliable information from controlled safety studies. The key elements of safety assurance include safety studies that examine the potential to cause both acute and delayed adverse biological outcomes, that determine the extent of exposure that can trigger those outcomes, and that establish standards that ensure identity and purity of the product.

Food Products

The main concern when the first food safety legislation was introduced in the early 1900s was that contamination by microbial or chemical contaminants from mishandling or intentional adulteration would result in the toxicity of a product that was inherently wholesome. Only more recently was it recognized that specific prospective testing is necessary to identify and quantitate the risks of serious conditions that require long periods to develop or that may occur only through interactions with other agents or in specific sensitive individuals.

Thus, the basic legislation that established food safety regulations in the period 1906 to 1938 focused on sanitation, proper handling and storage, manufacturing practices, and prevention of contamination. This focus has remained in the laws until the present time. Common foods do not require either premarketing or postmarketing safety testing, but are accepted as generally safe unless adulterated. This is significantly less rigorous than the requirements for extensive premarket testing of "new" (introduced after enactment of the controlling legislation) foods, food additives, pharmaceuticals, and pesticides. The FDA is empowered to take action against food containing harmful constituents (or the USDA in the case of meat, poultry, and egg products), but there is no requirement for experimental establishment of safety prior to marketing by the person or entity producing or selling the product.

Of course, certain plants and animals are known to contain poisonous chemicals, and the FDA has the authority to control the use of and/or exposure to any food that is poisonous or that has a poisonous constituent. The Food, Drug, and Cosmetic Act differentiates between potentially poisonous constituents that are naturally present in foods and those added intentionally during the production, processing, and handling of foods, placing a more lenient safety standard on chemicals that are natural constituents in the food. Specifically, adulterated food is not permitted, and the law defines adulterated food as follows:

"§ 342. Adulterated food

A food shall be deemed to be adulterated— **(a) Poisonous, insanitary, etc., ingredients**

(1) If it bears or contains any poisonous or deleterious substance which may render it injurious to health; but in case the substance is not an added substance such food shall not be considered adulterated under this clause if the quantity of such substance in such food does not ordinarily render it injurious to health."

The law then goes on to specify that food additives, pesticide residues, and animal drug residues shown to be safe are permitted, as well as defining conditions that result in unacceptable microbiological risk. This distinction between added and naturally occurring constituents is of course a practical consideration, because the chemical composition of foods is extremely complex and it would be impractical to hold the marketer of the product responsible for conducting extensive safety testing of all of the many chemicals that are present naturally in foods. In other words, even though the effect of any given chemical does not depend on whether or not it is present naturally, our protective laws are driven in part by practical considerations of what is economically feasible to require and partly by established notions of what is likely to be harmful.

To ensure uniformity of product quality and safety, the FDA has established standards of identity and quality for many products. It is noteworthy, however, that the law specifically excludes standards of identity or quality for fruits or vegetables, stating:

"No definition and standard of identity and no standard of quality shall be established for fresh or dried fruits, fresh or dried vegetables, or butter, except that definitions and standards of identity may be established for avocadoes, cantaloupes, citrus fruits, and melons. . . . Any definition and standard of identity prescribed by the Secretary for avocadoes, cantaloupes, citrus fruits, or melons shall relate only to maturity and to the effects of freezing."

The FDA recognizes that, in addition to the impracticality of conducting prospective toxicity studies on the multitude of potentially toxic chemicals present endogenously in foods, contamination with certain chemical substances is unavoidable. Thus, the FDA has established action levels and tolerances for substances known to be toxic or deleterious, but that cannot practically be avoided at low levels. These action levels and tolerances represent limits at or above which FDA will take legal action to remove products from the market. Where no established action level or tolerance exists, FDA may take legal action against the product at the minimal detectable level of the contaminant. The FDA has issued a number of guidances that establish these action levels for poisonous or deleterious substances in human food products. Examples of such chemicals for which FDA guidances (guidelines) have been established include acrylamide, dioxins, polychlorinated biphenyls, melamine, certain radionuclides, arsenic, a number of mold toxins, and others. These guidances and action levels mitigate the risk of adverse effects of chemical constituents of food that are known to have adverse effects at exposure levels above those that are permitted.

In addition to FDA's authority to take action based on potential deleterious effects, another important safeguard that helps assure safety, identity, and quality of food products are FDA-mandated labeling requirements. FDA can take legal action to have a food product removed from the market if it is determined to be misbranded. Among other criteria, a food is deemed to be misbranded if its labeling is false or misleading in any particular, if it is offered for sale under the name of another food, is an imitation of another food, or if its container is made, formed, or filled so as to be misleading. Further, labeling must conform to requirements for standards of identity, quality, pasteurization, and nutrient content.

In response to recent concerns about threats related to intentional adulteration, for example from radical terrorists, the Food Safety Modernization Act of 2011 introduced requirements for the development of vulnerability assessments and mitigation strategies to protect against intentional adulteration.

Food Additives and Color Additives

New food additives and color additives used in food cannot be used until a food additive petition is submitted and approved by the FDA. The safety of these products must be established before they can be sold under a set of guidelines published by the FDA (U.S. Food and Drug Administration, 2007). Food additives are defined by the FDA as substances whose intended use results, or may reasonably be expected to result, directly or indirectly, in it becoming a component of food or otherwise affecting the characteristics of food. Direct food additives are compounds that are added to food to achieve a technical effect (*e.g.*, emulsification, sweetening, preservation). Color additives are dyes, pigments, or other substances used to color foods. Indirect food additives, sometimes referred to as food contact chemicals, include substances used in the production, manufacturing, packing, processing, preparing, treating, packaging, transporting, or holding of food (*e.g.*, chemicals in product containers, can coatings, paper and paperboard, sanitizers, adhesives, etc.). All of the above require that data supporting their safety be reported to the FDA and be reviewed and approved before use is permitted. The testing requirements for these products are hierarchical, with the extent of testing required dependent on the chemical structure class of the agent and the magnitude of exposure to the agent when used in an approved manner. Those considered to be in the highest risk category must undergo comprehensive non-human testing comparable to that for new prescription drugs, whereas those in chemical categories known to be relatively safe or with very low levels of exposure may be permitted to undergo a more abbreviated battery of safety tests. Although human testing of the safety of food additives is not required, this is often done for agents in the higher risk category. The FDA provides specific guidelines that assure the scientific integrity of all phases of the required testing and the nonclinical studies must adhere to Good Laboratory Practice rules that require third-party monitoring and review of the studies. Upon review of the supporting scientific evidence, the FDA determines an acceptable level of use by applying safety factors (sometimes called uncertainty factors) that account for the uncertainties in extrapolating from the laboratory data to human risk in order to assure that a level of exposure that could cause harm is not reached.

Agents that had an extensive history of safe usage before passage of the FFDCA food additive amendment of 1958 or that have an extensive body of published literature that supports their safety are considered to be generally recognized as safe (GRAS) and are exempted from the food additive petition process. There is a formal procedure for submission and review of products that determines whether they can be granted GRAS status.

Overall the regulations and guidelines in place provide a high degree of safety assurance for these types of products.

Organic Food Products

Organic food products are a special class of products believed by many to be more nutritious, healthier, and safer than products produced by modern methods that employ pesticide application and/or the use of food additives to stabilize products and protect them from deterioration or microbial contamination. Being originally trained as a chemist, I feel obliged to point out that most chemicals present in foods are organic in the chemical sense, in that they are carbon-based chemical compounds. An organic chemist does not distinguish among organic molecules based on whether they are created by human chemists, living organisms such as plants and animals, or by natural environmental processes. However, the term "organic" used on a food product label in the grocery store has a special meaning under the law. According to the food labeling laws, an organic food product is one produced in accord with the provisions of the Organic Foods Production Act of 1990 (OFPA). The premise of the OFPA and the reason for development of the organic food market is the general belief that *synthetic* chemicals, made by man, are unhealthful, and that *natural* chemicals are inherently safer because they exist in nature. In the minds of many consumers committed to organic products, "chemicals" are viewed as those synthesized by man and those synthesized by plants are viewed as somehow different, and in particular less toxic.

The OFPA establishes standards governing the marketing and labeling of agricultural products as "organically produced products", and mandates the establishment of a system for certifying that farms and handling operations that produce food products claimed to be "organic" meet the standards of this Act. Under this law, to be sold or labeled as an organically produced agricultural product, the product shall:

1. have been produced and handled without the use of synthetic chemicals, except as otherwise provided in this law
2. not be produced on land to which any prohibited substances, including synthetic chemicals, have been applied during the three years immediately preceding the harvest of the agricultural product (except as otherwise provided in the act and excluding livestock)
3. be produced and handled in compliance with an organic plan agreed to by the producer and handler of such product and the certifying agent

As discussed earlier, the scientific evidence does not support the supposition that naturally occurring chemicals are necessarily safer than those synthesized by chemists. However, like DSHEA, the Organic Foods Production Act is clearly based on this general supposition. In this author's view, both laws suffer from the same "natural mistake" of assuming that health risk is associated primarily with man-made synthetic chemicals.

The OFPA and its associated regulations do not specify safety testing standards or establish premarketing safety testing requirements, but they do include a National List of Allowed and Prohibited Substances (commonly referred to as the National

List) that is developed and maintained by a National Organic Standards Board (NOSB). This list includes specific synthetic agents that are recognized as safe and specific non-synthetic agents that may be unsafe or undesirable. While this clearly provides a level of consumer protection, it is not the same level provided by the laws that require intensive prospective testing of synthetic pesticides or food additives for potential delayed and low-frequency, but serious and often life-threatening, health effects and the establishment of conservative safety margins for allowable exposures.

The OFPA created the NOSB to implement standards for organic food production, to develop the National List of Allowed and Prohibited Substances that can be used in the production of organic products, and to advise the Secretary of Agriculture on all aspects of the National Organic Program (NOP). The governing regulations are specified in U.S. Code of Federal Regulations (see references CFR Part 205, Subchapter M, Organic Foods Production Act Provisions), which contains criteria for determining which substances and ingredients are allowed or prohibited in products to be sold, labeled, or represented as "organic" or "made with organic (specified ingredients or food group(s))." The National List identifies specific substances that may or may not be used in organic production and handling operations of both agricultural crops and livestock. Synthetic chemicals may not be used in the production and handling of organically produced agricultural products unless such synthetic substances are placed on the National List. Thus, the National List includes both synthetic and non-synthetic substances.

Products meeting the conditions established may be labeled to indicate that the product meets Department of Agriculture standards for organic production and may incorporate the Department of Agriculture seal on its label. Imported products may be sold and labeled as organically produced if it is determined that the product has been produced and handled under an organic certification program that meets the standards of this law. The labeling regulations are somewhat confusing because there are four different categories of permitted labeling of organic products. Consumers should be aware of the meaning of the different wordings permitted to be used in the labeling. Products that contain *only* organically produced ingredients (excluding water and salt) can be labeled "100 percent organic" and can include the USDA seal. Products that contain at least 95% organically produced products (excluding water and salt) can be labeled "organic" and include the USDA seal as long as the percentage of organic ingredients is included and the ingredients that are organic are specified on the label. If a product contains less than 70% organically produced ingredients, the label may identify the specific organically produced ingredients as "organic" and display the percentage of organic content on the label but the USDA seal or the seal of any certifying agent may not be displayed. Products that contain at least 70% organically produced ingredients may be labeled "made with organic (specified ingredients or food groups)" as long as no ingredients are made using prohibited practices and may include the seal of a certifying agent but may not include the USDA seal.

Although imported organic products sold in the United States are required to meet the same standards as those produced in the U.S., a recent report by the Office of the Inspector General of the U.S. Department of Agriculture (USDA, 2017) identified deficiencies in assuring compliance of foreign imports. For example, imported agricultural products may be fumigated with pesticides at U.S. ports of entry to prevent the introduction of foreign pests into the U.S., but the USDA has not established controls to assure that these fumigated products are prevented from being sold as organic. The deficiencies identified in this report can result in the acceptance and sale of imported products labeled as organic that in fact do not meet organic standards.

A key question is whether organically produced food products are in fact more healthful and/or more nutritious than those produced using modern farming and processing methods that may include the use of synthetic pesticides. This, of course, determines whether the higher prices commanded by organic products are worth the additional expense. Chemicals synthesized by man and chemicals synthesized by plants may each have either low or high toxic potency. Since plants produce their own pest and disease deterrents, the prohibition of the use of well-studied synthetic pesticides and disease-prevention agents necessarily creates a strong incentive for the organic farmer to use those cultivars with the highest levels of these natural protective chemicals. This raises the question of whether organically produced products could be less safe than those produced by traditional methods. A further consideration is that insect and microbial attacks stimulate plants to increase the production of the endogenous secondary metabolites that serve to protect the plant, and therefore organically farmed products are more likely to have higher levels of these naturally occurring pesticides due to stress from attack by pests than those raised under conditions of systematic treatments used in conventional farming.

I do not argue that organically produced products are necessarily less safe or less healthful than conventional products, as there is a lack of evidence that this is the case. However, the converse statements, that organically produced foods are safer than conventional ones or that conventionally produced food is less safe and less wholesome than organically produced foods, are clearly false. The belief that organic foods are safer or nutritionally superior is not supported either by direct scientific evidence or by logical deduction based on consideration of the extent of available safety information and regulatory oversight of these two classes of products. It is important to recognize that the "natural mistake" embodied in the DSHEA and OFPA has resulted in the thoroughly studied and well-defined health risks of synthetic pesticides and food preservatives being replaced by unknown potential risks from naturally occurring defensive chemicals in plants and botanical supplements that are not well studied and in most cases are entirely unknown.

Like the DSHEA there is essentially no focus on premarket safety testing of the products and their constituents covered under the OFPA. It is also noteworthy that the CFR section that specifies the regulations implemented under the OFPA begins by defining "nontoxic" to mean "Not known to cause any adverse physiological effects in animals, plants, humans, or the environment". "Not known to cause adverse effects" is *very* different than "known not to cause any adverse effects". The pesticide and food additive laws are written with the intent to assure that studies of various potential toxicities must be conducted and safety verified before marketing is permitted. DSHEA and OFPA are based on the presumption that products can be assumed to be safe until the regulatory agency demonstrates actual, or a strong probability of, harm under conditions of use. Thus, there are two major deficiencies in the safety provisions of the OFPA and its associated regulations. The first is the preceding definition of nontoxic, which assumes that certain classes of chemicals are safe without specific prospective evidence that this is in fact the case. The second is the lack of consideration of whether the prohibition against using synthetic pesticides and preservative agents leads to increased risk from insect and microorganism resistant plant cultivars that contain unstudied natural pesticides and pest deterrents. Given the knowledge that plants have evolved to produce endogenous chemicals that convey resistance to insect and microbial attack (as discussed in chapter 2), it is highly likely that cultivars used for organic farming will contain higher levels of these natural pesticides than those that can be used with traditional farming techniques.

Although there is no substantive evidence that organic products present a significantly higher health risk than conventionally produced products, my point is that most people assume that organic products are more healthful but in fact there is no good evidence that this assumption is correct. On the contrary, there is not only reason to question the premise but reason to suggest that the focus of organic production—to eliminate risks that are already controlled to minuscule levels by the rigorous regulations controlling the use of pesticides and food additives—leads to the substitution of unknown health risks due to selecting and breeding more highly pest-resistant varieties that contain naturally occurring pest-resistance chemicals that are not required to be studied.

My personal conclusions are that 1) one mistake in this case is an economic one, in that there appears to be little or no basis for paying the cost premium associated with organic production, and 2) there should be a revision of the health and safety laws that provides a more uniform balance of evaluation of potential risks from both natural and man-made sources.

Genetically Modified Food Products

The safety of genetically modified foods (GM foods) or a genetically modified plant or animal, referred to as a genetically modified organism (GMO) or bioengineered food (BE food), is regulated in the United States under the legislation that governs the particular product in question. Thus, genetically modified organisms may be regulated by more than one regulatory body or by more than one division of a major regulatory body. For example, GMO-derived foods are regulated by the FDA Center for Food Safety and Applied Nutrition, GMO-derived drug products by the FDA Center for Drug Evaluation and Research, and GMO-derived biological products by the FDA Center for Biologics Evaluation and Research. GMO pesticides are regulated by the EPA under the FIFRA. Genetically modified animals are regulated by the FDA Center for Veterinary Medicine. Genetically modified plants are regulated by the USDA under the Plant Protection Act and the Agricultural Marketing Act. And so on. The FDA has in place a voluntary consultation process through which producers of new genetically engineered food plants can consult with the FDA regarding the safety of foods derived from the new plants. Specific premarketing safety testing requirements have not been established and premarket review of safety studies is not required, but this voluntary process is relied upon to resolve any safety issues that may impact the FDA's regulatory actions with regard to the product. Genetically modified animals used as foods must be evaluated for safety of the food product, effectiveness of the genetic modification for achieving the desired result (*e.g.*, enhanced or more rapid growth), for lack of adverse effect on the animals themselves, and absence of adverse effects on the environment (U.S. Food and Drug Administration, 2017).

Modern methods of genetic manipulation have made modification of the genetic makeup of organisms more precise and more efficient in comparison with conventional methods of breeding and selection of new plant cultivars. Genetic modification through selection of specific cultivars with particular characteristics, crossbreeding to establish desirable genetic traits, and mutagenesis followed by selection of desirable characteristics have long been used to modify the expression of genes that affect the content of biochemical products that confer favorable characteristics or eliminate unfavorable ones (Wikipedia, 2018). Virtually all current plant crops have undergone extensive genetic manipulation through conventional breeding and selection processes to increase yield, increase disease and pest resistance, reduce toxicant levels, and/or to improve nutrient content. One of many examples is the development of the currently used canola oil, which is widely marketed in the U.S. and other countries. The current product is derived from the seeds of *Brassica* species of plants originally known as rape or rapeseed that have been selected and manipulated to reduce the content of the anti-nutrient and toxicant erucic acid and to modify the content of saturated fatty acids to optimize the nutritional quality. The history of this development is succinctly presented in an OECD document on compositional considerations for new varieties of low erucic acid rapeseed (canola) (OECD, 2011). In spite of consumer worries about genetic manipulation using modern molecular methods, these older methods generally introduce more unknown genetic changes than do the more specific modern molecular engineering methods.

In addition to the introduction of genetic alterations by such human interventions, the transfer of genetic elements into plants from other organisms can also occur naturally. For example, bacteria known to be pathogenic to plants, such as *Agrobacterium rhizogenes* and *Agrobacterium tumefaciens*, are known to exchange fragments of their DNA into plants. Crown gall disease, often found in orchards and vineyards, is known to be caused by the transfer of part of a plant tumor-inducing plasmid from the *Agrobacterium tumefaciens* bacterium into the plant genome. These DNA fragments are biologically active and result in the formation of a class of chemicals called opines in the infected plant. Recently it was found that these types of DNA fragments occur in cultivated sweet potatoes, demonstrating that these food plants are naturally transgenic (*i.e.*, that they contain fragments of DNA from the bacteria that have become integrated into the plant genome (Kyndt *et al.*, 2015)). Thus, natural modification of the DNA of plant foods occurs in nature, and is not specific to human genetic manipulation.

The application of modern genetic methods that allow specific modification of specific targeted genes is relatively recent. Unlike the traditional methods of selection and crossbreeding, that introduce large numbers of uncharacterized genetic modifications with unknown biochemical functions in addition to those that produce the desirable trait that is sought, the newer biochemical methods have become very specific and allow changes to be made at will in single genes with known functions.

The first approved commercial genetically engineered food crop was the FLAVR SAVR tomato, which was introduced in 1994. This plant was engineered to suppress the expression of a gene that produces an enzyme (polygalacturonase, PG) responsible for dissolving a cell wall component of the tomato (pectin), thereby allowing the ripened fruit to remain firm longer. This allows the tomato to be vine ripened to a more advanced stage without softening to a degree that prevents transportation to the marketplace. The result is development of more favorable flavor and transportation characteristics. Suppression of the production of the PG enzyme was achieved by introducing a reverse-oriented copy of the native gene that dramatically reduces the formation of the native enzyme by reducing the level of the RNA molecule that codes for synthesis of this protein. Although this product appeared to be accepted when first introduced, it eventually failed to be commercially successful—in large part due to unsubstantiated consumer concerns about safety that led to discontinuance of sales by some large retail outlets (Bruening and Lyons, 2000).

The importance of GM crops has increased dramatically since the introduction of modern methods of genetic manipulation. As examples of the economic importance of GM crops, in 2013 93% of soybeans, 90% of cotton, and 90% of corn grown in the U.S. were genetically engineered for either herbicide resistance or insect resistance (Law Library of Congress, 2014). Relative to some other countries, the U.S. laws governing GM foods and other GM products are less restrictive, and this is probably a factor contributing to the fact that the U.S. is the world's leading producer of GM crops.

The AquAdvantage Salmon was the first genetically engineered animal approved for food use in the U.S. This salmon, which was approved for food use in 2015, contains a gene for salmon growth hormone that results in accelerated growth. It was approved by the FDA under a New Animal Drug Application. This required premarket demonstration of the safety of the food product, the effectiveness of the modification for improving production of the fish, evaluation of adverse effects on the fish, and an environmental assessment that evaluated potential adverse effects on the environment if the fish were to escape from the breeding facility. Given the effectiveness of genetic engineering, it can be expected that genetically modified food products will continue to play an expanding role in effective food production.

In addition to GM plants and animals used as foods, the FDA has regulatory authority over genetic modifications of non-food animals. Such genetic modifications are considered to be animal drugs, and hence are regulated by the FDA Center for Veterinary Medicine. One of the first non-food genetically modified animals introduced into commerce was the GloFish, an aquarium fish into which have been incorporated genes from marine organisms that produce highly fluorescent molecules that cause the fish to glow in fluorescent colors under ultraviolet or other light. The first of these was a modified zebrafish. In 2003 the FDA determined that since aquarium fish were not used for foods and therefore did not pose a risk to the food supply, and since there was no evidence that the genetically engineered fish posed any greater threat to the environment than did their unmodified counterparts, the FDA concluded that there was no reason to regulate these particular fish. These fish are now widely available in U.S. pet stores, along with aquarium tanks and fluorescent accessories for use in conjunction with displays of the fluorescent fish (see Wikipedia article that summarizes the history of their development, <ins>https://en.wikipedia.org/wiki/GloFish</ins>).

There is a general consensus among regulatory scientists that genetically modified foods are as safe and nutritious as conventional foods. For example, a report by a committee of the U.S. National Academies of Sciences, Engineering, and Medicine (2016) concludes:

"On the basis of detailed examination of comparisons of currently commercialized genetically engineered with non-genetically engineered foods in compositional analysis, acute and chronic animal toxicity tests, long-term data on health of livestock fed genetically engineered foods, and human epidemiological data, the committee found no differences that implicate a higher risk to human health from genetically engineered foods than from their non-genetically engineered counterparts."

Similarly, a report of the scientific Council of the American Medical Association (2001) states that no long-term health effects have been detected from the use of transgenic crops and genetically modified foods, and that these foods are substantially equivalent to their conventional counterparts. The Food and Agriculture Organization of the United Nations concludes:

"Currently available transgenic crops and foods derived from them have been judged safe to eat and the methods used to test their safety have been deemed appropriate. These conclusions represent the consensus of the scientific evidence surveyed by the ICSU (International Council for Science, 2003) and they are consistent with the views of the World Health Organization (WHO, 2002) . . . To date no verifiable untoward toxic or nutritionally deleterious effects resulting from the consumption of foods derived from genetically modified crops have been discovered anywhere in the world (GM science review panel). Many millions of people have consumed foods derived from genetically modified plants – mainly maize, soybean, and oilseed rape – without any observed adverse effects (ICSU)."

The American Association for the Advancement of Science (AAAS) Board of Directors in 2012 issued a report that states:

"The main conclusions to be drawn from the efforts of more than 130 research projects, covering a period of more than 25 years of research and involving more than 500 independent research groups, is that biotechnology, and in particular GMOs, are not per se more risky than e.g. conventional plant breeding technologies."

The Society of Toxicology, the largest scientific society for professionals that evaluate product safety and chemical and product hazards and risks, issued a statement in November 2017 concluding that there has been no verifiable evidence of potential adverse health effects during the 20-year period since genetically engineered crops have been approved for use (Society of Toxicology, 2017). They conclude that genetically engineered crops have been a major economic success, have greatly improved farming efficiency, and have helped reduce or maintain overall food costs. Their position statement recognizes that some scientists and many consumers continue to be concerned about the potential for unrecognized risks from GM food crops, but emphasizes that conventional breeding methods that use naturally occurring genetic variation or breeding strains intentionally mutated by non-specific means to induce desirable traits introduce far more unknown genetic alterations. They note that modern genetic engineering techniques that introduce only a highly specific and well-characterized alteration are far more precise. Importantly, products of the more modern genetic engineering techniques generally undergo more extensive evaluation of the quality and safety of the resulting product than do those of traditional breeding methods. The Society of Toxicology report concludes: "*to date, such studies have not revealed any evidence that foods from GM crops present a risk for adverse health or nutritional effects, but have helped demonstrate overall suitability based on the species of the crop.*"

Other reviews by scientists and national and international organizations support these conclusions. Of course, some articles can be found that express concerns about possible safety issues and others that correctly point out that the nature of genetic engineering is such that each new genetically modified product needs to be evaluated on a case-by-case basis to be sure that some unique feature of a particular construct does not present an unanticipated health concern. The same is true of conventional breeding and selection of natural genetic variants for particular traits. The overall consensus is that safeguards currently in place in developed countries make genetically modified plants and plant products at least as safe as their conventional counterparts.

Despite these scientific assessments, there are still concerns about genetic modification. Aside from specific health issues related to genetic modification of food crops, acceptance or non-acceptance of these modified products can have very significant economic consequences. A prime example of this is the case of Viptera corn which was developed and marketed by Syngenta AG, one of the largest agricultural seed and agrochemical producers in the world. This corn was bioengineered to contain genes from a soil bacterium that confer resistance to a number of pests, including earworms, cutworms, corn borers, and armyworms as well as other pests such as molds. The proteins produced by these genes are toxic to the pest species but are digested by animals and have been shown to be nontoxic in toxicology studies. Viptera corn seeds were approved for sale in the U.S., Canada, and Japan in 2010, were introduced to the U.S. marketplace in 2011, and were widely planted in that year. In 2013 China, which had not yet approved this genetically modified corn variety, began rejecting imports of corn containing this variety. Because corn shipments generally include corn produced from many different fields, corn shipments that contained even small amounts of Viptera corn were rejected by China. This has led to thousands of lawsuits against Syngenta, claiming that the company is responsible for losses of billions of dollars in the corn market because they did not obtain approval from China to accept the product before selling and marketing the seeds for this corn. The suits claim that even farmers that did not grow Viptera corn suffered losses because of the rejection of shipments in which the various types of corn were co-mingled in grain elevators and/or shipments and therefore rejected. China subsequently granted import approval of Viptera corn in December of 2014, but only in 2017 did the first of these cases come to trial (*Naples Daily News*, 2017). This case, involving multibillion-dollar consequences, illustrates the economic magnitude and the extended timeframes of impacts associated with the use of genetically modified crops.

Interestingly, a recent survey by the Pew Research Center (Funk and Raine, 2015) shows that the largest difference between opinions of the general public and scientists associated with the American Association for the Advancement of Science (AAAS, a group representative of U.S. scientists) is their view of the safety of genetically modified foods. Although 88% of surveyed AAAS scientists considered genetically modified foods safe to eat, only 37% of U.S. adults shared this opinion. This survey also shows that individuals more highly educated in science have much greater confidence than the general population in the safety of genetically modified products. This is also true of the level of confidence in the safety of pesticide residues allowed in foods (68% of AAAS scientists considered foods grown with pesticides safe to eat, whereas only 28% of U.S. adults shared that opinion). Although the percentage of scientists surveyed who expressed reservations about the safety of foods grown with pesticides (32%) was higher than those expressing concern about the safety of genetically modified foods (12%), this higher level of concern about the safety of pesticides is very likely due to the fact that this particular survey did not distinguish between the disciplines of the scientists surveyed, and most of those surveyed were likely unfamiliar with the highly conservative methodology used to establish allowable safe levels of pesticides in food products.

For readers interested in delving further into the topic of the safety of genetically modified food products, Wikipedia presents a well-referenced and balanced discussion of the safety of genetically modified foods (see https://en.wikipedia.org/wiki/Genetically_modified_food). The searchable FDA website (www.fda.gov) also contains much relevant information on this topic.

The preceding discussion is not to say that there cannot be safety problems with genetic engineering. One notable incident that illustrates the type of problem that can occur is the

"ProdiGene incident". This case is succinctly described in an internet posting by the Federation of American Scientists (https://fas.org/biosecurity/ education/dualuse-agriculture/2.-agricultural-biotechnology/prodigene-incident.html) and in an article by Ellstrand (2003). This is a case in 2002 in which a biotechnology firm named ProdiGene Inc. was producing a pharmaceutical product in a genetically modified agricultural crop (corn), and the genetically modified corn, containing a biologically active pharmaceutical agent (avidin, a biotin-binding protein), was inadvertently co-mingled with a subsequent food crop. The company involved, ProdiGene, was conducting field trials with the modified corn that produced the protein avidin intended for diagnostic applications, and then the same field was replanted with soybeans. The field contained leftover kernels of corn that germinated and then grew into plants that were co-harvested with the soybean food crop and became co-mingled. This was discovered and the company was ordered to destroy 500,000 bushels of soybeans intended for food use in veggie burgers and infant formula. The company was also fined $250,000 by the USDA for failing to follow the required procedure for assuring that such co-mingling did not occur and the company had to pay more than three million dollars in addition for the costs of quarantine and destruction of the soybean crop. In another incident with the same company, a field of corn used for pharmaceutical production cross-pollinated with a neighboring field, resulting in the destruction of 150 acres of possibly contaminated plants.

Another case is that of StarLink corn (https://fas.org/biosecurity/education/dualuse-agriculture/2.-agricultural-biotechnology/starlink-corn.html). In this case, a transgenic variety of yellow corn, called StarLink corn, was approved by the U.S. EPA in 1998. This corn variety had been genetically engineered to contain a gene for *Bacillus thuringiensis* (Bt) that produces a toxin that kills destructive corn borer larvae, and it was approved only for use as an animal feed because of the potential for an allergic response to the Bt toxin. However, genes from the StarLink corn were detected in taco shells and other corn food products, demonstrating that the corn had been co-mingled with conventional corn. This resulted in recalls of food products found to contain the bioengineered corn and led to the withdrawal of the license for production of this variety of corn. Other types of corn engineered to produce pesticidal metabolites have been extensively tested for toxicity and allergenicity, found to be safe, and continue to be produced.

Although the violations in these cases were caught and corrected, the cases illustrate the potential for untoward incidents that could have adverse health consequences. As a result of these incidents, increased attention is being focused on rules that prevent cross-contamination between food and non-food crops, and new genetic varieties undergo extensive testing. Thus, as is the case with all product types, regulatory oversight with careful production controls are essential if an optimally safe food supply is to be assured.

Pesticides and Pesticide Residues in Food

Pesticides and pesticide residues in foods are regulated by the Environmental Protection Agency under the Federal Insecticide, Fungicide, and Rodenticide Act (FIFRA) (U.S. Environmental Protection Agency, 2017). Before a manufacturer can sell a pesticide in the United States, a pesticide registration must be obtained. This requires an in-depth series of studies that establish the chemical characteristics of the product, form the basis of an assessment of potential human health effects and environmental effects, and establish its biological performance against the target pests. The chemical characterization includes establishing the product identity and purity, characterization of impurities, stability studies, a method for its chemical analysis, and more. Health effects studies include comprehensive acute, repeated dose, and chronic toxicity tests as well as studies of reproductive, carcinogenic, neurotoxic, and mutagenic potential, and studies of metabolism and elimination. Environmental effects studies include effects on non-target organisms in laboratory and field tests, along with studies of applicator exposure, spray drift evaluations, environmental fate, and more.

If the pesticide is to be used on a food product, the above requirements of a pesticide registration must first be met and registration (*i.e.*, a license that permits sale of the pesticide) obtained and then the EPA will establish a residue tolerance. The tolerance is the permissible amount of residue that may remain in a food product. In some countries these are called maximum residue limits. If residues above this level are found, the product is subject to seizure by the government. Tolerances are very conservative, and take into account the toxicity of the pesticide and its break-down products, how much remains in the food after various application regimens, consumption levels of foods on which the pesticide may be used, and other possible sources of exposure to the same pesticide or other pesticides with similar biological activity. After considering these and other factors, safety margins are applied to ensure consumer protection.

After a tolerance has been established, the FDA monitors food products to ensure compliance with the residue limits, the USDA tests milk and meat, and both agencies maintain databases of residues that are found and share this information with each other and the EPA to ensure that safe levels are being maintained.

Although many consumers believe that natural pesticides in disease-resistant plants are preferable to the use of the pesticides offered by commercial pesticide producers, these natural pesticides are not necessarily safer than synthetic ones. Since pesticides marketed by commercial producers under FIFRA requirements must undergo the extensive safety testing, careful documentation of their purity and identity, and are routinely monitored for the maintenance of safe levels in products, whereas endogenous pesticides associated with disease-resistant plants and natural products not approved under FIFRA requirements do not require any testing at all (nor is documentation and control of the purity and identity of the endogenous pesticides required) there is little apparent logic to assuming that these latter classes are safer and more environmentally sound choices. Indeed, logic indicates the opposite—careful study of potential health effects coupled with regulatory oversight and market basket surveys to assure that guidelines are being followed so that conservative levels of safe exposure are not exceeded make conventional products developed under FIFRA requirements the more rational choice.

"Natural" Food Products

Given the extensive consumer interest in natural products and the ubiquitous use of the term "natural" in product advertising and on product labels, not to mention the use of this term in the title of this book, one may wonder why "natural products" have not yet been discussed at the same level of detail as the other topics of this chapter. Although one might assume that this term would be clearly defined in the laws and regulations governing the production and marketing of foods, dietary supplements, and other consumer products, surprisingly this term has never been clearly defined in FDA regulations or in the food and drug laws. Thus, the definition of a "natural" food product as it is applied to the marketing and labeling of products remains ambiguous. This lack of a clear definition is likely to change in the near future, as several pending lawsuits and citizens' petitions submitted to the FDA have pushed the Agency to undertake a regulatory guidance to clarify the issue of the use of the word "natural" in product labeling and advertising. As of June 2017, this guidance has apparently not yet been completed. In the meantime, the FDA has posted its current regulatory position on a webpage that addresses the use of the word "natural" on food labeling. In part, this webpage (www.fda.gov/food/food-labeling-nutrition/use-term-natural-food-labeling) states:

"Although the FDA has not engaged in rulemaking to establish a formal definition for the term "natural," we do have a longstanding policy concerning the use of "natural" in human food labeling. The FDA has considered the term "natural" to mean that nothing artificial or synthetic (including all color additives regardless of source) has been included in, or has been added to, a food that would not normally be expected to be in that food. However, this policy was not intended to address food production methods, such as the use of pesticides, nor did it explicitly address food processing or manufacturing methods, such as thermal technologies, pasteurization, or irradiation. The FDA also did not consider whether the term "natural" should describe any nutritional or other health benefit."

On this webpage, the FDA asked for comments from the public and industries on questions such as:

- *Whether it is appropriate to define the term "natural,"*
- *If so, how the agency should define "natural," and*
- *How the agency should determine appropriate use of the term on food labels.*

The comment period closed May 10, 2016, and 7690 comments have been received by the FDA. Many of these comments suggested that any GMO product should not be referred to as natural, and some felt that only food products that met the organic food criteria should be allowed to claim that the product is natural. Until a more specific guidance or a final ruling is issued by the FDA, uncertainties will remain regarding the meaning of this term when used on a food label. In particular, clarification with regard to the allowance of minor residues of chemicals used in production, processing, or packaging; the use of various processing methods; genetic modification of crops; or selective breeding practices that enhance or suppress specific natural components of the product is needed. Additionally, although the FDA is finally addressing the use of this term on food products, personal care and cosmetic products are also frequently described as "natural" and the labeling requirements for those products will also require further clarification.

Finally, aside from the question of whether a product labeled as "natural" is truly unaltered by human intervention, let us not lose sight of the more important question. That question is whether those products that are produced entirely by nature are inherently safer than those produced or modified by humans. As has been discussed at length, the scientific evidence strongly indicates that no meaningful generalization can be made on this point. Both man-made and naturally occurring chemicals have been shown to have a wide range of human health effects, with many chemicals from each of these classes being extremely toxic, many others largely without any significant biological effects at exposure levels encountered under actual living conditions, and others providing nutritional benefits or medicinal value in the treatment of diseases and pathologies. Only careful and thorough studies of these biological effects, and knowledge of the relationship between exposure level and effect of each chemical constituent, can define the safety and health benefits of any specific chemical or product.

Concluding Comments

The federal laws discussed apply to the sale of products in interstate commerce, and individual states also have laws that apply to production, sale, and use within those states. Food additives, color additives, and pesticide residues are more tightly regulated than foods, because the former require prospective premarket testing prior to sale (with the exception of food additives "grandfathered" as safe due to their widespread use prior to the adoption of the controlling legislation in 1958). Contrary to widespread belief, there is no requirement that the FDA or the EPA test the safety of any regulated products, and little actual testing of products is carried out by these agencies. For those products that require testing prior to marketing, the company or person selling the product must perform the testing. For those products with a premarketing testing requirement, the Sponsor (company or person wishing to sell the product) is required to obtain and submit to the regulatory agency the experimental data necessary to establish the safety (and in the case of food additives, also efficacy) of the product for its intended use. Thus, the burden of "proof" of safety and/or efficacy of these products is on the Sponsor and the regulatory agency serves as the judge of its adequacy. The FDA is given the authority to prevent the sale of, or to seize, unsafe food products, but neither the FDA, the producer or manufacturer, nor the seller is required to perform safety testing of common foods. The FDA and EPA have never been expected to perform, nor have received the budget allocations that allow them to perform, comprehensive routine testing of the safety or efficacy of marketed products.

Chapter 9

Regulation of Dietary Supplements, Pharmaceuticals, and Cosmetics

Botanical Supplements: A special case under the law

The regulatory requirements for the marketing and advertising of dietary supplements, including "nutraceuticals" and other botanical dietary supplements that are marketed to "promote health", are in stark contrast to the requirements for the rigorous testing of new food additives, prescription drugs, and pesticides prior to allowing them to be sold. Dietary supplements are regulated by the Dietary Supplement Health and Education Act of 1994 or DSHEA and can be sold without any requirement for such premarket testing as long as they don't contain new dietary ingredients that were not marketed prior to October 1994. The DSHEA defines the term "dietary supplement" to mean a product (other than tobacco) intended to supplement the diet that is or contains one or more of the following dietary ingredients: a vitamin, a mineral, an herb or other botanical, an amino acid, a dietary substance for use by man to supplement the diet by increasing the total dietary intake, or a concentrate, metabolite, constituent, extract, or combination of any of the aforementioned ingredients. This law explicitly states in Sec. 2.:

"Congress finds that–

(14) dietary supplements are safe within a broad range of intake, and safety problems with the supplements are relatively rare; and

(15)(A) legislative action that protects the right of access of consumers to safe dietary supplements is necessary in order to promote wellness."

In other words, without scientific data to support the claim, Congress has declared that dietary supplements are inherently safe and that safety problems are relatively rare—thereby codifying into law the great mistake (in my scientific opinion) that botanical supplements, even if concentrated, are to be considered safe without the need for safety testing or of approval by the FDA prior to their sale! The FDA website on dietary supplements points out that firms are prohibited under the DSHEA from marketing products that are adulterated or misbranded, and therefore are responsible for evaluating the safety and labeling of their products before marketing. Manufacturers must also register their facilities with the FDA. However, there is no requirement for specific premarket safety testing and so the burden of proof that a product is in fact adulterated rests in large part on the FDA. Likewise, although manufacturers are required to register their facilities, they are not required to obtain FDA approval prior to producing or selling dietary supplements.

Importantly, dietary supplements marketed to "improve or support health" are in fact often used with the intention of preventing, or even mitigating or curing, disease, but are not subject to the stringent requirements or regulations that would apply if a disease prevention, mitigation, or cure claim were made. Unlike the case of prescription pharmaceuticals, dietary supplements may make claims regarding health benefits as long as they include on the product label a statement (that may be in a relatively small font) that states that the health claims have not been evaluated by the FDA. A product sold to "promote organ health" is in effect being used to reduce the risk of developing diseases of that organ, but is not subject to the premarket testing requirements or establishment of rigorous identity standards that would be required under the Food, Drug, and Cosmetic Act if this intent were stated explicitly.

The testing and documentation of the study observations required of pharmaceutical agents results in reports of all adverse effects in the tests conducted, and this information must be made public. This allows marketers of "nutraceutical" products to tell customers that many toxic effects have been observed with the pharmaceutical product. Unfortunately, in most cases dietary supplements and "nutraceuticals" have not undergone the same rigorous testing that would reveal high-dose adverse effects, and so potential high-dose adverse effects and the safety margin between these effects and the exposure from product usage are unknown. This is one of the principal causes of the erroneous perception that natural botanical supplements are "safer" than conventional pharmaceutical products—a perception that is often enhanced by marketers of botanical supplements who claim that their products can promote health without the known "side effects" of conventional pharmaceuticals. Also of importance is that dietary supplement advertising is regulated by the Federal Trade Commission (FTC) and not by the FDA, although the FDA does regulate the labeling of the product. The FDA and FTC do attempt to coordinate their oversight responsibilities, but the FTC does not have the same depth of expertise in the biological sciences as does the FDA.

The misconception that natural and botanical products are safer than conventional pharmaceuticals is not borne out by scientific studies. In addition to the many known acutely toxic plant constituents, large-scale testing programs for longer-term effects such as cancer show that natural and man-made products contain similar proportions of agents that produce adverse health effects. For an excellent discussion of the acute and chronic effects of natural and synthetic chemicals, see the public access article by the well-known biochemist Dr. Bruce Ames and his colleagues in the *Proceedings of the National Academy of Sciences* (Ames *et al.*, 1990).

New dietary ingredients are treated differently than supplements marketed prior to the passage of DSHEA in 1994, in that a notification of intent to market a product containing, or consisting of, a new dietary ingredient must be filed with the FDA 75 days prior to offering it for sale. Premarketing approval by the FDA is still not required, but the notice provides information about the identity and safety of the new ingredient and allows the FDA the chance to raise concerns or objections prior to the product being offered on the market.

DSHEA defines a new dietary ingredient (NDI) as:

"a dietary ingredient that was not marketed in the United States before October 15, 1994, and does not include any dietary ingredient which was marketed in the United States before October 15, 1994."

and specifies that:

"A dietary supplement which contains a new dietary ingredient shall be deemed adulterated under section 402(f) unless it meets one of the following requirements:

(1) The dietary supplement contains only dietary ingredients which have been present in the food supply as an article used for food in a form in which the food has not been chemically altered.

(2) There is a history of use or other evidence of safety establishing that the dietary ingredient when used under the conditions recommended or suggested in the labeling of the dietary supplement will reasonably be expected to be safe and, at least 75 days before being introduced or delivered for

introduction into interstate commerce, the manufacturer or distributor of the dietary ingredient or dietary supplement provides the Secretary with information, including any citation to published articles, which is the basis on which the manufacturer or distributor has concluded that a dietary supplement containing such dietary ingredient will reasonably be expected to be safe."

What this means is that ingredients in dietary supplements that were in use before the passage of the DSHEA in 1994 can be marketed without notifying the FDA, but that the FDA must be notified of the intent to market a supplement containing a dietary ingredient that wasn't already marketed as an ingredient in a supplement before this date. This notification must provide evidence in the notification to justify the conclusion that the ingredient is reasonably expected to be safe. As stated in the above text from the law, published articles can be used to support the reasonable expectation of safety. Until relatively recently, there were no detailed specifications of the types of safety studies that should be used to evaluate the safe use of an NDI. Currently, the FDA is preparing a guidance on new dietary ingredients that does specify types of study data that would support the required expectation of safe use and that should be included in an NDI notification. Within 75 days of receipt of an NDI notification, the FDA would respond with a letter that either acknowledges receipt without objection or that lists deficiencies or safety concerns. In the latter cases the FDA could ask for further information, or, if safety concerns were sufficient, could conclude that the ingredient would be considered an adulterant. Although the DSHEA was passed in 1994, this guidance was still not final as of early 2019 although a comprehensive draft was issued for comment in 2011 and was updated in August 2016.

In conjunction with the draft guidance on new dietary ingredients, the FDA has undertaken development of an authoritative list of ingredients exempt from this notification requirement. The director of the FDA Office of Dietary Supplement Programs has indicated a willingness to work with "stakeholders" (marketers of products, customers, and other interested individuals) in the development of this list. This is expected to be a difficult and time-consuming process. There is an existing compendium entitled *Herbs of Commerce* published by the American Herbal Products Association but the FDA draft guidance makes clear that they are unlikely to regard this compendium as "solely determinative" of whether an ingredient qualifies for exclusion from the filing requirement.

When fully implemented, this FDA guidance will bring the "requirements" (FDA guidances are not legally binding, but set forth FDA expectations that are generally followed by product Sponsors) into much closer alignment with those for new food additives. In the meantime, 1) supplements and dietary ingredients marketed in the U.S. prior to October 1994 may be marketed without FDA notification or approval, 2) supplements and dietary ingredients not marketed in the U.S. prior to October 1994 may still be marketed without FDA approval but require FDA notification 75 days prior to offering it for sale of intent to offer the product for sale and the basis for the marketer's conclusion that it is safe, and 3) there is no official listing of those products considered exempt from the premarketing notification requirement, leaving it up to the marketer of the product to determine whether the premarket notification is necessary.

Pharmaceutical Products (Human Drugs)

Pharmaceutical products are regulated by the Food and Drug Administration. Prior to being sold, new prescription medications must undergo a comprehensive set of biological tests in both laboratory studies and human clinical trials to evaluate their mechanism of therapeutic action, to determine their potential to cause adverse health effects, and to demonstrate that they are clinically effective. Importantly, in addition to evaluating the potential for acute toxicity (toxicities that occur shortly after exposure to the product) the potential for causing delayed or difficult to detect effects such as cancer induction, delayed neurological effects, behavioral effects, and reproductive effects must be rigorously evaluated prior to the product being allowed to be sold. Additionally, manufacturing standards that assure consistent identity and purity must be established and the safety of impurities must be proven. Individual states also have safety laws, but in most cases federal requirements are at least as rigorous as state laws.

Because drug products are a direct source of biologically active chemicals and have a history of drug-related toxicities, it should not be surprising that this is the most tightly regulated and thoroughly tested class of consumer products. The Federal Food, Drug, and Cosmetic Act (FFDCA) defines a drug as an article intended for use in the diagnosis, cure, mitigation, treatment, or prevention of disease in man or other animals. This definition is important because many dietary supplements are in fact sold and used to prevent disease but are exempted from the extensive testing required for a drug product because the Dietary Supplement Health and Education Act (DSHEA) allows exclusion from these requirements as long as they are advertised and labeled only with the claim that they "promote health" rather than prevent or cure disease.

In the case of a drug, the extensive program of laboratory and human clinical testing that is required to demonstrate that the product is both effective and safe includes investigations of the absorption, distribution, and metabolism of the drug, the concentrations of the drug in blood and tissues, and verification of the function and integrity of essentially all important organ systems in the body. This includes assessment of reproductive function, microscopic evaluation by a certified pathologist to verify the integrity of all important tissues in the body, measurements of cellular composition and levels of biomarkers that indicate either tissue damage or normal organ function (similar to the blood work performed in a comprehensive physical examination by doctors), and documentation of the state of health, growth, and behavioral function in both laboratory animals and human studies. These studies are conducted in at least two relevant animal species using exposures of various lengths and including dose levels that include the expected therapeutic level and also higher doses that cause adverse effects. The higher dose level testing allows setting of safety margins that assure that the approved doses do not cause toxicity. There are also special studies of fetal development, of growth and behavior of newly born offspring, evaluation of the potential to cause genetic damage, studies of behavioral effects in adult animals, of effects on the immune system, and finally studies of lifetime exposure that include assessment of toxic and cancer-causing potential.

The laboratory studies reveal the expected adverse effects that must be monitored in human studies to verify the safety of the levels proposed for clinical use. They also establish the expected time courses of effects, the metabolic pathways by which the drugs are altered in the body, and the molecular mechanisms of both beneficial and adverse effects in mammalian species that have been selected to model these same effects in humans. In addition, studies of effects in cell cultures provide further information about the effects on normal cell metabolism and function. All of these studies are conducted under strict Good Laboratory Practices and Good Clinical Practices guidelines that require an independent third party to check compliance with approved study protocols and to verify the accuracy of data and calculations.

A noteworthy aside to the regulatory policies designed to assure the safety of pharmaceutical products is that even when a natural product is clearly classified as a pharmaceutical agent it may still be exempted from certain of the rigorous testing requirements that apply to a synthetic drug product or active ingredient. For example, pharmaceutical agents have strict testing guidelines that require the assessment of the potential for impurities to have the capacity to cause damage to DNA, which is believed to be an indicator of their ability to cause cancer. This guideline, entitled *Assessment and Control of DNA Reactive (Mutagenic) Impurities in Pharmaceuticals to Limit Potential Carcinogenic Risk,* was recently updated in March 2018 (FDA, 2018). Importantly, this guidance document specifically excludes herbal drug products or crude products of plant origin from these important safety testing requirements that apply to synthetic drug products, stating: *Assessment of the mutagenic potential of impurities as described in this Guidance is not intended for the following types of drug substances and drug products: "... (other classes) ... herbal, and crude products of animal or plant origin."* One might ask if there is a sound scientific basis for this exclusion. Given that natural plant sources of biologically active chemicals that have proven useful as drugs usually have many structurally related chemicals with biological activities, it might be more logical to ask why the requirements for naturally occurring mixtures should not be *more* rigorous than those for specific synthetic chemicals rather than less!

Comprehensive animal and cell culture studies are followed by rigorous human clinical trials that are conducted "double-blind", meaning that neither the doctors conducting the study and evaluating the results nor patients receiving the drug are aware of whether the patient received a placebo or the drug. This assures that the expectations of the patients and the doctors do not bias the results of the study. These studies are very tightly controlled and require the rigorous documentation of all adverse health effects in the subjects being studied as well as careful documentation of disease status and progression. Health assessments include those normally conducted in comprehensive physical examinations, and include assessment of blood cell composition and plasma or serum biomarkers of normal and abnormal organ function and tissue damage, ECGs, specialized health studies applicable to the disease state of the population being treated, and expected therapeutic and adverse effects. One important difference from the preclinical testing for health effects is that tests for cancer induction and reproductive performance are not generally conducted in humans because the technical requirements for the conduct of such studies in humans are not regarded as ethical and therefore the conduct of such studies is prohibited. Therefore, protection against these types of effects relies almost exclusively on the findings in animal studies.

In addition, regulations require the methods of chemical synthesis of the drug to be established and tightly controlled, the drug's stability under storage conditions determined, and its impurity profile defined and impurity limits specified. All impurities above a certain level must be identified and verified safe, and analytical identity standards must be established and carefully documented, reviewed, and approved by the FDA, then subsequently monitored during production, distribution, and use of the drug. Additionally, after approval of the drug, there is an adverse event reporting system through which physicians, patients, and other health care providers are encouraged to report to the FDA any adverse effects suspected to be associated with the use of the product. The FDA reviews these reports on an ongoing basis and may use this information to issue product warnings, request safety studies from Sponsors, or to implement regulatory actions.

All of this testing must be meticulously documented by following rigorous government guidelines for nonclinical and clinical study conduct and reporting, and all of the above information must be reviewed and approved by the FDA, usually with recommendations from external expert advisory committees, prior to receiving approval to market (sell) the drug product. Key findings from these studies are summarized in the "drug label", which is made available to physicians and pharmacists authorized to prescribe and dispense the drugs and also made available to the patient in a somewhat less technical format.

Over-the-counter drugs (OTC drugs) have slightly different regulatory requirements than prescription drugs, although the safety and efficacy requirements of both classes are substantially the same. The Durham-Humphrey Amendment of 1951 formally differentiated drugs into two classes, prescription drugs and over-the-counter drugs. This amendment of the FFDCA requires that drugs that are habit-forming or potentially harmful must be dispensed under the supervision of a health practitioner as a prescription drug and must carry the statement, "Caution: Federal law prohibits dispensing without a prescription." OTC drugs may be approved either through the normal new drug application process used for prescription drugs or by a monograph process described in the Code of Federal Regulations (21 CFR 330).

Under the latter process a panel of experts evaluates the safety and efficacy data available, reviews the proposed drug labeling, and advises on promulgation of a monograph that establishes conditions under which the OTC drug is recognized as safe, effective, and not misbranded (designated GRASE, for **g**enerally **r**ecognized **a**s **s**afe and **e**ffective). Relevant information is solicited *via* the Federal Register, the expert panel makes recommendations to FDA for establishment of a monograph, public comments on the panel's recommendations are solicited, and after consideration of the panel recommendations and comments received the FDA may then establish a final monograph that specifies conditions under which the proposed OTC drug is safe and effective. The types of data reviewed by the expert panel are essentially the same as those required for prescription drug approval. The main differences between the new drug application process for OTC drugs and the monograph process is that the former is a confidential process specific to a particular drug product that may permit marketing exclusivity. The monograph process is a public process with a central role of an external panel of experts that establishes acceptability of an active ingredient with no potential for marketing exclusivity.

Given the rigorous requirements for the conduct, reporting, and review of prospective safety and efficacy testing and for establishment of detailed standards of identity, purity, and manufacturing processes for new drugs, it is ironic that the consumer perception is more often than not that pharmaceutical products are less safe than botanical supplements. Scientific facts and judgment support the opposite conclusion.

Cosmetics

Cosmetics are another class of product that does not require approval before sale in the U.S. There are two principal laws that regulate interstate sales of cosmetics, the Federal Food, Drug, and Cosmetic Act and the Fair Packaging and Labeling Act. The regulations established under these laws are administered by the FDA. Cosmetics are defined in the Food, Drug, and Cosmetic Act as *"articles intended to be rubbed, poured, sprinkled, or sprayed on, introduced into, or otherwise applied to the human body . . . for cleansing, beautifying, promoting attractiveness, or altering the appearance."* Such products include skin moisturizers, shampoos, hair colors, deodorants, lipsticks, perfumes, fingernail polishes, etc.

The law states that the marketing of adulterated or misbranded cosmetics in interstate commerce is prohibited, but the burden of proof to establish adulteration or misbranding is on the FDA. A product is considered adulterated if it contains any poisonous or deleterious substance that may render it injurious to users under the conditions of use prescribed in the labeling, or of customary or usual use, if it contains unsanitary, filthy, or putrid components, if its container is composed of constituents that may be injurious to health, or if it contains a color additive that is unsafe. Misbranding includes a product with false or misleading labeling, a label that does not include all required information, that has a container formed or filled so as to be misleading, or that has packaging or labeling in violation of the Poison Prevention Packaging Act of 1970. A product may also be considered misbranded due to failure to provide material facts, for example, directions for safe use or warning statements needed to ensure safe use.

As is the case with dietary supplements, the FDA has the authority to pursue enforcement action against products not in compliance with the law or against firms or individuals that violate the law. Companies and individuals who manufacture or market cosmetics have a legal responsibility to ensure the safety of their products, but there are no specific tests required to demonstrate the safety of products or ingredients. Further, there is no requirement that cosmetic companies share safety information they may have with the FDA. There is a system of cosmetic ingredients review by panels of recognized experts that is relied upon by the FDA to critically evaluate the safety of cosmetic ingredients. However, the burden of proof of health risk or other types of noncompliance with the law is on the FDA and the FDA must substantiate such risk or noncompliance in order to take regulatory action.

In addition to the FDA's limitations with regard to its ability to assure cosmetic product safety, a further major issue with respect to cosmetics safety is the European Cosmetics Regulation that prohibits animal testing of cosmetic products sold in the European Union. Since most major companies are multinational, most large companies are being forced to test cosmetic products using *in vitro* test methodologies that may not be reliable predictors of certain important types of toxic responses. Although essentially all regulatory scientists ascribe to the principle of minimal use of animal testing when possible, the current consensus among most regulatory toxicologists is that animal testing is still required to provide protection against many important types of harmful effects. These include cancer induction, neurological effects, and reproductive effects, which are of concern especially for products with constituents that are absorbed through the skin. Even the European law that bans such testing acknowledges that non-animal tests currently do not adequately assess some important toxicities, such as repeated-dose toxicity and reproductive effects, and that *in vivo* toxicokinetic behavior cannot be adequately determined in non-animal tests.

Many consumers opposed to animal testing specifically choose cosmetic products that are advertised to be produced without animal testing, believing that adequate safety assessment is currently possible without animal testing. In many cases such advertising is misleading because many products are advertised as not being tested in animals when the final product has not been tested in animals but the ingredients in the product have in fact previously been proven safe through animal testing. However, in the case of ingredients that have actually never been tested in animals, consumers are placing themselves and their family members at the risk that certain important types of potential toxicity may be undetected. In essence, the consumer and family members that purchase and use such untested products are the test subjects for these types of toxicity.

Concluding Comments

In summary, provisions for safety assurance are not uniform among different products. Foods, drugs, cosmetics, dietary supplements, and pesticides each have different regulatory requirements and oversight. Foods with a long history of use and cosmetics do not have to be tested for safety prior to their sale. Food additives in use prior to the 1958 food additives amendment and dietary supplements in use prior to the 1994 Dietary Supplement Health and Education Act of 1994 may also be marketed without preapproval by the FDA. New food additives, pesticides, and drugs must undergo extensive testing prior to being sold in interstate commerce. For those products that require testing prior to marketing, the Sponsor (company or person wishing to sell the product) is required to submit to the regulatory agency the experimental data necessary to establish the safety (and also efficacy in the case of pharmaceuticals and food additives) of the product and to obtain approval of the regulatory agency prior to offering it for sale. Regulatory oversight is complex, with different divisions of the FDA, USDA, EPA, and FTC responsible for oversight of different products and aspects of their production, manufacturing, sale, labeling, and advertising.

Critical factors in product safety assurance are the extent of safety testing data that is available for evaluation and whether the burden of "proof" of safety, health risk, and/or efficacy of these products is on the Sponsor or on the responsible regulatory agency. For those products that may be marketed without regulatory approval, the burden of proof of harm, or unreasonable risk of harm, is on the regulatory agency and products can remain on the market until such harm or unreasonable risk is established. Those products that are generally perceived by the public as presenting the greatest health risk, pesticides, food additives, and prescription pharmaceuticals, are not only those with the most substantial evidence of safety, but are those for which evidence of safety and methods for assuring product identity and purity must be established and implemented prior to being sold. These products therefore have a relatively low potential for unanticipated harm, as any safety problem is likely to have been identified before consumers have been exposed.

Chapter 10

Burden of Proof: A Critical but Under-Appreciated Factor in Product Risk

One of the most important but least appreciated factors that determine the degree of consumer safety assurance is whether the legal framework that governs a product's safety requirements places the burden of proof to demonstrate product safety on the company or individual manufacturing or selling the product, or whether the burden of proof to demonstrate harm or risk of harm is on the regulatory agency responsible for oversight of the product's safety. As has been discussed, for some products the company or individual producing or selling the product (the product Sponsor) must demonstrate that it is safe based on a prospective safety testing program before it is allowed to be sold. In other cases, the burden is on the responsible regulatory agency to demonstrate that a particular product is harmful to the consumer under the conditions of product use after it is being marketed before regulatory action can be taken. When the regulatory agency has the burden of proof to demonstrate harm, there is a general provision that the company or individual selling the product should have evidence of product safety prior to selling it but there is often no requirement that such evidence be submitted to the FDA. Further, for products that do not require specific premarket testing, it is generally accepted that a history of use without reported adverse effects is sufficient evidence of safety—and the fallacy of this assumption should be evident from the examples presented in earlier chapters.

If the company selling the product is not required to conduct specific safety testing and the FDA does not review and evaluate the evidence of safety or efficacy prior to sale, the level of safety assurance is generally low and depends in large part on the voluntary responsibility taken by the product Sponsor. Even when the FDA has a cause for concern, it usually does not have either the funding necessary to perform the highly expensive testing required to meet the standard that would be applied to the Sponsors of those products that must establish safety prior to marketing or sufficient authority to require the same degree of testing by the Sponsor. Regulatory agency resources tend to be disproportionally allocated to those products for which the Sponsor is required to conduct safety testing and to obtain review and approval from the agency before the product may be sold. Areas such as investigation and follow-up studies of adverse event reports related to botanical supplements receive fewer resources, even though it is obvious that the public would benefit from increased emphasis on this data-poor class of products.

The pharmaceutical, food, and agrochemical industries and their lobbyists want, and lobby for, FDA and EPA resources to be directed at rapid review of required studies and expect prompt responses to submitted applications because they are barred from marketing their products until FDA or EPA approval has been received. In the case of the botanical and health food industry the incentives are the reverse—because companies are allowed to sell their products without any requirement to submit data that could result in marketing restrictions, their incentive is to minimize FDA attention on their products because that could potentially limit the marketing of products that are already being sold.

The imbalance of resources devoted to evaluation of the safety of different classes of products is extreme. For example, according to a report issued in November 2014 by the Tufts Center for the Study of Drug Development, the average capitalized cost of the research and development programs conducted by industry in order to bring one novel new pharmaceutical agent to market was at that time greater than 2.5 billion dollars. This includes the costs of the laboratory research necessary to identify promising drug candidates, to establish documented production methods that assure standardized product identity and purity, to conduct laboratory regulatory studies necessary to demonstrate safety and potential efficacy prior to initiating clinical trials, and to conduct and submit reports of blinded human clinical trials that demonstrate the safety and effectiveness of the drug use under the conditions of clinical use. This also includes the costs associated with developmental agents that fail to reach the market. Similarly, the cost to conduct the necessary studies and to register a new pesticide was estimated to be approximately 256 million dollars during the period 2005-2008, and is undoubtedly greater now (Bunge and McKay, 2017). In contrast, botanical supplements that have been marketed prior to 1994 can be sold without any required safety or efficacy testing.

In addition to the industry costs, the cost to the government associated with the review of the studies of those products requiring premarket agency approval is also extremely high. It might be thought that the government regulatory agencies responsible for product safety would devote more resources to those classes of products that can be sold without premarket testing and for which they have the burden to identify and substantiate health-related issues than to those classes that are required to be thoroughly tested by the companies before sales are allowed. In fact, the latter classes have far more government regulatory resources devoted to them. Overall, the annual FDA budget is approximately 5.4 billion dollars with more than 17,000 full-time staff. Of this, in 2018 the FDA Office of Dietary Supplement Programs (ODSP) had only 26 full-time-equivalent staff and was expected to have an operating budget of approximately 7.3 million dollars with which to regulate dietary supplement product safety. In comparison, the drug and biologics medicines review and approval programs employed more than 6500 full-time staff and had a budget of more than two billion dollars. The foods program had approximately 1000 full-time staff and received 1 billion dollars, and the animal drugs and feeds program had 596 staff and received 198 million dollars. Thus, the dietary supplements regulatory program is grossly underfunded relative not only to the programs with oversight of the more rigorously controlled human drugs, foods, and food additive products, but even with respect to the animal feeds and drugs programs.

The FDA Center for Food Safety and Applied Nutrition has the principal regulatory responsibility for dietary supplements safety, but until recently the priority afforded this area of responsibility has been relatively low. For example, the 2015 budget justification submitted to the congressional appropriations committees, which summarizes the priorities of the foods and veterinary medicines programs (U.S. Food and Drug Administration, 2014), does not even mention the dietary supplements component of the program, stating: *"The mission of the Foods and Veterinary Medicine Program is to protect and promote the health of humans and animals by ensuring the safety and proper labeling of the American food supply, animal feed, and cosmetics, as well as the safety and effectiveness of animal drugs and devices."* The fact that the dietary supplements program was not considered of sufficient priority to warrant mention in this introductory statement of the mission goals that support the budget request reflects the relatively low priority of the dietary supplements program compared to other agency programs. However, under

Commissioner Scott Gottlieb the dietary supplements program recently received a higher priority. In contrast to the 2015 budget request, the overall program mission statement included with the 2020 budget request (U.S. Food and Drug Administration, 2019) reads: "*The purpose of the Foods Program is to protect and promote human health by ensuring the safety of the American food supply, dietary supplements* [underline added for emphasis], *and cosmetics, as well as the proper labeling of food and cosmetics.*". This indicates the increased priority this component of the program is now receiving. Nonetheless, the dietary supplements program continues to receive only a small fraction of the FDA's resources.

In the case of dietary supplements, the FDA has the burden of conducting or financing at least some of the expensive laboratory studies necessary to evaluate safety in order to determine if there is a substantial basis to initiate regulatory action when existing literature reports are insufficient to support safety or spontaneous reports to the FDA of adverse reactions suggest a need for further studies. Given current staffing, with less than 30 staff and a budget of approximately 7.3 million dollars in the FDA Office of Dietary Supplement Programs involved with the regulation of dietary supplements, it is simply not possible to address safety issues adequately. This level of funding would not allow even one product per year to be tested according to the standards required of pharmaceuticals, food additives, or pesticides. Thus, the FDA cannot provide a comparable level of safety assurance of supplements regulated under the DSHEA. In recognition of this fact, the FDA requires that retail botanical supplement products be labeled to state that health claims made by the company have not been evaluated by the FDA. Only the most extreme cases of toxicity or health risk can be expected to be evaluated by the FDA.

Even when a significant product-related toxicity related to a dietary supplement has been identified, the hurdles faced by the FDA when attempting regulatory action are substantial. In addition to the examples already presented, the story of

1,3-dimethylamylamine, or DMAA, is another illustration of the difficulties faced by the FDA when attempting regulatory action against harmful dietary supplements (Welsh, 2013; U.S. Food and Drug Administration, 2013). DMAA is a chemical that was developed as a nasal decongestant drug by the Eli Lilly Company in the 1940s. It is a derivative of amphetamine, and it was removed from the market in 1983 at the company's request after studies had shown increases in heart rate, blood pressure, nervousness, and tremors. However, in the mid-2000s it became widely used as an active ingredient in performance-enhancing and weight loss supplements. It was often advertised as a natural derivative of geranium. As this use increased, reports of deaths and illness, including cardiovascular problems, shortness of breath, and heart attack linked to DMAA accumulated. After six deaths and more than 100 reports of illness were linked to DMAA, including the deaths of four soldiers at Fort Bliss, all apparently healthy and taking DMAA as a performance enhancer, the FDA banned DMAA in April 2012.

In response to the military cases, the defense department conducted a study of 2000 active-duty personnel and found that more than 15% of those surveyed were taking DMAA and 40 had reported illness after taking the supplement. Two soldiers in this group suffered liver failure. By 2012, the military and several other countries including Canada, the United Kingdom, and New Zealand had banned or restricted the use of DMAA. In 2012 the FDA issued warning letters notifying companies selling products with DMAA as an ingredient that the products needed to be removed from the market or reformulated to remove DMAA.

Although most companies complied with the FDA request, USPlabs, which sold the popular products OxyElite Pro and Jack3d, did not. This company continued to manufacture and sell these products containing DMAA, arguing that it stood behind the safety and quality of its products and citing a number of peer-reviewed reports of clinical studies that it claimed established the safety of its products. In May of 2013 the Texas Department of State Health Services stepped in and embargoed the product at the USPlabs warehouse in Dallas, Texas. Then, the FDA used its authority under the Federal Food, Drug, and Cosmetic Act to detain the USPlabs' products, which were subsequently turned over to them by the Texas State authority. Under this authority, the FDA can detain a dietary supplement product if it has reason to believe the product is adulterated or misbranded, but this authority only allows them to keep it out of the marketplace for a maximum of 30 days while it determines if further action, such as seizure, is warranted. USPlabs initially challenged the FDA's conclusion that DMAA was unsafe, but after the FDA issued a formal response letter notifying the company that it did not agree with its position and that removal of the DMAA-containing products was needed they agreed to voluntarily destroy the detained product, valued at more than eight million dollars.

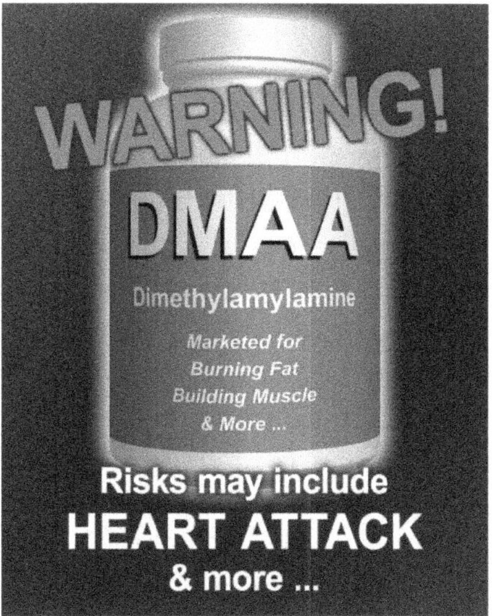

Figure 10.1 DMAA warning from FDA website (see FDA, 2013)

But the story does not end there. After finally agreeing to withdraw DMAA-containing products, USPlabs then reformulated OxyElite Pro, without changing its name, to contain aegeline in place of DMAA (*Dallas News*, 2013). Aegeline is an extract of the bael tree, and this new formulation has been linked to fatal liver disease. In one report, more than 60 people were reported to be sickened including two who required liver transplants and a mother of seven in Hawaii who developed liver failure and died after taking the new formulation to lose the weight she had gained during pregnancy. The FDA then determined that aegeline was an illegal ingredient and issued a warning letter to the company that resulted in voluntary withdrawal of the new formulation.

However, this is still not the end of the story. In November of 2017, after DMAA and aegeline were determined by the FDA to be illegal ingredients, Dr. Pieter Cohen of Harvard Medical School and colleagues bought six online products being marketed as weight loss or pre-workout exercise products to check for DMAA analogs and found four chemically- and pharmacologically-related chemicals, including DMAA itself (Schultz, 2017). Thus, this case clearly illustrates the continuing limitations of the FDA's powers to implement regulatory action against products regulated under DSHEA in a timely fashion and also confirms the common practice of companies to simply change the formulation and re-introduce modified products when an FDA warning is issued or other regulatory action is taken.

Because the burden of proof to demonstrate harm in order to take regulatory action against unsafe botanical supplements lies with the FDA, products often remain on the market for extended periods after adverse effects have been identified while data is obtained and analyzed to establish the basis for regulatory action, warnings are issued and contested, and/or legal action implemented. After such action is finally taken, companies will often then voluntarily withdraw the product, reformulate it, and return it to the market with another ingredient that may create a new safety issue, requiring the FDA to repeat the cycle and again build a scientific case that supports a new regulatory action. This is in marked contrast to the situation with food additives, pesticide residues, or pharmaceutical agents, which are not permitted to enter the marketplace until comprehensive studies that establish their safety and, when appropriate efficacy, have been completed and found to be satisfactory by the responsible regulatory agency.

Chapter 11
Avoiding "Toxic" Chemicals: The Exploitation of Confusion Between Toxic Hazard and Risk of Toxicity

It is common to think of chemicals as being either safe or toxic. This perception underlies the widespread practice of avoiding all foods that contain chemicals perceived to be toxic, such as chemical additives and pesticide residues. Unfortunately, it is not this simple. Everything in the world is composed of chemicals, and most chemicals can be toxic at some exposure level but are nontoxic at lower exposure levels. It is simply not possible to categorize chemicals as being either safe or toxic without taking into account the degree of exposure to that chemical because the risk of toxic effects depends on both the toxic potency of the chemical and the degree of exposure that occurs.

It is important to understand that potential adverse biological effects can be identified only by understanding the relationship between toxic potency and the extent of exposure that occurs in real-life situations. The process of determining this relationship is referred to as *risk assessment*. The first component of risk assessment is the determination of the type of adverse effects that can be induced by exposure and the exposure levels at which they occur. This is determined either experimentally by testing a range of higher and higher exposure levels until a toxic effect occurs, or by analysis of human data that show the exposure levels associated with known adverse effects. This component of risk assessment is referred to as *hazard identification*. The next component of risk assessment is the determination of the relationship between exposure (or dose in the case of drugs or dietary supplements) and the toxic response, or *exposure-response assessment*. Subsequently the expected toxic outcomes that could result from the exposures in actual use and higher possible accidental exposures are considered, referred to by some agencies as *risk characterization* or simply *risk assessment*. This includes identification of exposure levels that do not cause the identified effects and takes into account potential exposures and uncertainties in extrapolating the available data to the human exposure situation. This then allows an assessment of safe *vs.* harmful levels during actual product use and as a result of other levels of exposure. The final step, *risk management*, is the process of using the available data to minimize or eliminate any potential risks and includes control measures that assure that allowable risks are not exceeded.

The more thoroughly a particular substance has been studied the more likely it is that some toxic effect will have been identified at very high exposure levels. Thorough study also makes it far more likely that the levels allowed in a given product are based on a well-established safety margin that assures a *lack* of toxicity under conditions of normal product use. Unless specific safety studies have been conducted to provide the information needed for a meaningful risk assessment, the lack of reports of toxicity can never be assumed to assure product safety. This critical distinction between *hazard* (the potential to cause a certain type of toxicity if an exposure is sufficiently high) and *risk* (the probability that the potential toxicity will actually occur at a given exposure level) lies at the heart of the science of toxicological evaluation and safety assessment.

It is debatable whether product marketing that points to high-exposure effects out of context is a deliberate scare tactic designed to deceive the consumer or simply a result of misunderstanding the critical difference between toxic hazard and risk of toxicity and the methodology used by regulatory scientists to assure safe products. Undoubtedly, each explanation applies in particular cases. Whichever is the case, consumers need to understand this difference in order to evaluate the relative safety of different products. The key principle of risk determination is that the combination of the level of exposure and toxic potential determines toxicity and not toxic potential alone. Credit for first articulating this principle is generally given to the Renaissance physician Paracelsus who wrote in the early 16th century that "*all substances are poisons; there is none which is not a poison. The right dose differentiates poison from a remedy.*" As a physician, Paracelsus was applying this statement primarily to medicinal drugs, but because it is generally true of any chemical exposure this quotation appears in the introduction to most general toxicology textbooks. It is unfortunate that the two critical concepts encompassed in the above statements are not taught to all students at an early age, because a clear understanding of the principles of hazard and risk is necessary to make informed decisions related to all types of risks encountered in daily life. This same principle applies not only to health risks, but more broadly to all forms of cause and effect.

The key underlying principles of health risk that everyone should understand are: 1) that a hazardous substance is something with the potential to cause harm, and 2) the risk that a hazardous substance will actually cause harm depends on whether a sufficient level of exposure is reached. In the more general sense, the risk of any particular outcome depends on the potency or magnitude of the causative factor and the extent of exposure to that factor. So, for example, a high-voltage electrical line presents the hazard of death by electrical shock, but the risk of anyone receiving a fatal shock from any given electrical line depends on the extent of exposure to the electrical voltage and current carried by that line. There is a negligible risk that your child walking to school will be harmed by the electrical lines contained safely in conduits buried under the street or from lines suspended from electrical towers. Likewise, one can safely use an electrical appliance with properly insulated electric cords, but the risk of receiving a fatal electrical shock is great if you use your hair dryer while in the bathtub or if you walk through a puddle into which an uninsulated high-voltage wire has fallen. In other words, it is the combination of the hazard of the electrical current carried by the high-voltage wire and the extent of probable exposure to that hazardous current that determines the risk of an adverse effect (such as fatality) due to exposure to the hazard. This same principle applies in essentially all cases of risk assessment. It is relatively meaningless to ask if it is safe to let your child cross a road unless this question is accompanied by information about the nature of the road and the level of traffic on it. No one would allow their child to cross a Los Angeles freeway during rush hour, but most would have no problem allowing them to cross a country road closed to automobile traffic that ran adjacent to their house. This same principle applies to other forms of cause and effect. For example, a high-powered automobile engine running at maximum speed has the potential to rapidly accelerate an automobile, but this will only occur if the power of the engine is transferred to the wheels that actually move the automobile.

In the case of chemical toxicity, the risk of toxicity from a particular chemical depends on the ability of the chemical to cause a particular type of toxicity, the potency of the chemical to cause these effects, and the extent of exposure of the particular organ or tissue that is susceptible to the toxic effect of that chemical. Thus, a highly potent liver toxicant is a toxic hazard, but the degree of risk it presents depends not only on its toxic potency but also on the extent of exposure of the liver to the chemical. Ingesting that chemical may not be a risk if it is not absorbed from the gut and transferred to the liver. Both benefit and harm always depend on the intrinsic toxic and beneficial properties of the chemical, its toxic or beneficial potency, and the extent of exposure to the organ or tissue that is affected. A meaningful assessment of these factors can be made only when appropriate human data are available or laboratory studies at high doses are conducted to allow determination of the types of toxic effect that can occur, the tissues and organs that are susceptible to those effects, and the exposure levels at which those effects occur. If one does not understand the above principles and the methods used to determine safe levels of constituents in consumer products, misleading health claims suggesting that products lacking the data needed to assure safety are safer than those for which comprehensive studies have established a far greater level of safety assurance are likely to be accepted.

In the case of a chemical that has a benefit, in addition to levels associated with toxic effects the exposure level that confers the desired benefit must also be taken into account. This requires the determination of both an exposure that is virtually always safe and the lowest dose that gives the desired beneficial effect. In the case of medicinal drugs, the ratio between these two levels is referred to as the "*therapeutic ratio*" or "*therapeutic index*" or sometimes the "*safety margin*" for that drug. For classes of drugs with the same therapeutic benefit those with the highest therapeutic ratio (*i.e.*, greatest difference between the beneficial and toxic exposure levels) will be the safest because toxicities are highly unlikely to occur at or even above therapeutic dosages. In the case of food additives, such as chemical antioxidants that protect against spoilage and rancidity, only chemicals with very large margins between the level needed for the desired effect and the level that might cause toxicity are permitted, and the level permitted to be used is the minimum required to produce the desired effect.

In the case of medicinal drugs, food additives, and pesticide residues, these safe levels and safety margins are required by law to be determined prior to the sale of products containing them. In the case of naturally occurring food constituents such as antioxidants, naturally pest-resistant food plants, or botanical dietary supplements, those products may be sold without the testing necessary to determine these safe levels and safety margins—and therefore serious potential toxicities may not have been identified and safety margins are often unknown. It is paradoxical that many consumers believe these latter classes are the safer, and unconscionable that the marketers of the latter classes use the absence of critical safety data to infer to customers that their products are safer than the former!

One might ask why consumers are particularly risk-averse when considering certain minimal health risks but readily accept other far greater and firmly substantiated risks. It is clear that factors other than rational scientific analysis have a major impact on consumer perceptions and practices. We have considered some of the reasons the negligible risks from food additives, pesticide residues, and GMO foods have led many consumers to avoid all products that contain them. But how can people rationalize the acceptance of risks such as continuing to smoke cigarettes when this is known to be responsible for 90% of male and 80% of female lung cancers, the highest single cause of cancer-related death for both men and women in the U.S.? The principles of risk assessment in both cases are identical, in that the risk depends on the extent of exposure and the potency of the identified hazard. The difference in perception seems to depend in part on an individual's personal experience with the hazardous element and therefore their confidence that personal knowledge and actions will minimize risk, in part on the perceived benefit from the practice in question, and in part on the degree of understanding of the actual risks involved.

If the average person were told that they needed to purchase an insulated suit to protect them from electrical hazards walking down the block from their home, the proposal would be perceived as ludicrous because the person would recognize that there was essentially no chance of exposure to the current carried by the electrical wires around their home. On the other hand, that same person might avoid foods containing the well-studied antioxidant food additives BHA or BHT, for which safety margins have been carefully determined and safe levels set by regulatory authorities. Further, that same person might purchase açaí berries for the perceived benefit of their high content of antioxidant chemicals, not recognizing that the phenolic antioxidants in açaí berries have chemical properties similar to the antioxidant food additives BHA and BHT but that have not been studied in a way that allows potential toxic effects and safety margins to be determined. These are inconsistent and illogical interpretations of relative risk, and are due in large part to the above factors.

Even regulatory agencies sometimes lose sight of the differences in their degree of acceptance of risks for different products. One example is the FDA's policy of accepting a history of use of new dietary ingredients without adverse health reports as acceptable evidence of safety when delayed effects, low-frequency events, and effects that depend on interaction with secondary factors would not be evident without specifically designed studies. Although this same agency is also responsible for the safety of foods and drugs, in the case of those products they require prospective quantitative evaluation of the risk of these same types of events before allowing them to be sold. These differences are not scientifically consistent but are a matter of policy determined by the legal framework.

Another reason for possible confusion about categorical classification of toxic *vs.* nontoxic chemicals is that in some cases products are required to be labeled as toxic, poisonous, or dangerous based on their toxic potency. This may seem inconsistent with the above argument that only the combination of toxic potency and extent of exposure determines the risk of toxicity.

However, in these cases the requirements are based on the assessment that the toxic potency of the product is sufficiently high that exposures large enough to cause toxicity could reasonably be expected to occur from exposure to the packaged product. For example, the Federal Hazardous Substances Act requires precautionary labeling on containers of hazardous household products to help consumers safely store and use those products, and to provide information about first aid steps to take if an accidental exposure occurs. This Act also allows the Consumer Product Safety Commission to ban certain products that have a toxic potency so high that the labeling the Act requires is not adequate to protect the consumer. If a product is toxic to laboratory rats at an exposure of 50 mg of product per kilogram body weight, which is equivalent to about 1/10 of an ounce to a 130-pound person, it is considered "highly toxic" and must be labeled with the word "poison". Similarly, the Department of Transportation requires products classified as toxic or poisonous materials, defined as a material so toxic to humans as to afford a hazard to health during transportation, or presumed to be so toxic to humans on the basis animal toxicity test results, to be labeled as "poison" or "toxic". Although these requirements are based on toxic potency, they are in fact a risk-based labeling requirement because a product of the specified potency presents a significant risk of an exposure sufficient to cause damage under the conditions of expected use or during transportation. This does not mean that any small exposure to the product presents a significant risk, but only means that direct exposure to the packaged product may be harmful. Unfortunately, many people mistakenly believe that substances are either toxic or safe, and that any exposure to a toxic substance may be harmful. In fact, almost any substance may be harmful if exposure is sufficiently high and, conversely, will be safe if exposure is sufficiently low.

Another risk of botanical products that contain complex mixtures of chemicals is that they may contain chemical constituents that are sufficiently toxic to cause harmful effects if extracted or concentrated. The Dietary Supplement Health and Education Act allows extracts of botanical supplements to be sold without a requirement for safety testing and does not specifically require separate testing of different mixtures of plant parts or of plants grown under different conditions of plant stress that might lead to increased exposure to specific chemical constituents. This leaves the potential for inadvertently increasing the concentration of specific chemical constituents that otherwise would have been safe, or selecting plant parts with higher concentrations, resulting in levels that would then prove harmful. In this way, exposure to minor constituents that are not normally toxic under conditions of historical use could reach harmful levels.

Chapter 12

What Really Matters:
Healthy Dietary and Lifestyle Factors
That Make the Most Difference

There is no question that a healthy diet is a critical lifestyle factor that has a favorable impact on our health. However, it is not the avoidance of residues of food additives and pesticides that have been proven to be the most important for optimal health. Rather, it is the positive influence of properly balancing intakes of essential macronutrients, vitamins, and minerals and avoidance of excess intakes of those dietary nutrients that have clearly been shown to have negative health impacts if intakes are too high. Control of sodium, saturated fat, added sugars, and total calories is especially important. Although much attention has been focused on the potential benefits of avoiding chemical food additives and pesticide residues, in fact there is little, if any, reliable evidence of any significant health benefit of an organic diet relative to consumption of conventionally farmed and produced foods. The scientific evidence shows that maintenance of a proper dietary balance of fat, carbohydrate, salt, and vitamin and mineral intake, along with maintenance of a healthy body weight and adequate exercise and sleep, are far more important.

There is overwhelming evidence that unbalanced diets high in saturated animal fats, salt, or sugar and carbohydrates, or deficient in adequate vitamins and minerals, as well as obesity, result in large increases in serious disease and death. Focusing on assuring appropriate intakes of fats, carbohydrates, fruits and vegetables, and fiber is of far more benefit than worrying about extensively studied and well-controlled additives and pesticide residues that have not been shown to have any significant adverse effects at permitted usage levels. Among the factors we can personally control, an appropriately balanced diet, maintenance of an appropriate body weight, and adequate exercise and sleep are the most important contributors to a long and healthy life. Of course, it is also important to avoid obvious detrimental behaviors such as smoking, excessive alcohol intake, and recreational drugs—and also poorly controlled botanical supplements, especially the frequently adulterated weight loss, athletic performance, and sexual enhancement classes.

Although not the primary focus of the present discussion, it seems important to consider some of the evidence that has identified the major factors that can improve our health and reduce the incidence of important diseases. The major health benefits of maintaining an appropriate diet are well-documented scientifically. Every five years the U.S. Departments of Health and Human Services (HHS) and of Agriculture (USDA) jointly evaluate the currently available scientific information and update the U.S. *Dietary Guidelines*. These *Guidelines* are required to be based on the preponderance of available scientific and medical knowledge, and they contain nutritional and dietary information and guidelines for the general public and professionals in the health care community. The latest edition (2015-2020) is available at <u>http://health.gov/dietaryguidelines/2015/guidelines/</u>. The guidelines are based on the *Scientific Report of the 2015 Dietary Guidelines Advisory Committee* and include consideration of comments received from federal agencies and the public. They are widely considered to be highly authoritative and are used in developing federal food, nutrition, and health policies and programs, as well as for federal nutrition education materials for HHS and USDA education programs that provide dietary and nutritional guidance.

This report concludes that: "*About half of all American adults have one or more <u>preventable, diet-related chronic diseases</u>, including cardiovascular disease, type 2 diabetes, and overweight and obesity.*" (Underlining added for emphasis.) The guidelines are based on the scientific evidence that a healthy eating pattern can minimize these preventable diseases. They are not a rigid prescription, but are an adaptable framework within which individuals can enjoy foods that meet their personal, cultural, and traditional preferences and fit within their budgets. Readers are strongly encouraged to access the *Dietary Guidelines*, to review the full report in detail, and to follow their recommendations. Key recommendations from these guidelines follow:

The Dietary Guidelines' *Key Recommendations for healthy eating patterns should be applied in their entirety, given the interconnected relationship that each dietary component can have with others.*

Consume a healthy eating pattern that accounts for all foods and beverages within an appropriate calorie level.

A healthy eating pattern includes:

- *A variety of vegetables from all of the subgroups—dark green, red and orange, legumes (beans and peas), starchy, and other fruits, especially whole fruits*
- *Grains, at least half of which are whole grains*
- *Fat-free or low-fat dairy, including milk, yogurt, cheese, and/or fortified soy beverages*
- *A variety of protein foods, including seafood, lean meats and poultry, eggs, legumes (beans and peas), and nuts, seeds, and soy products*
- *Oils*

A healthy eating pattern limits:

- *Saturated fats and trans fats, added sugars, and sodium*

  Key Recommendations that are quantitative are provided for several components of the diet that should be limited. These components are of particular public health concern in the United States, and the specified limits can help individuals achieve healthy eating patterns within calorie limits:

- *Consume less than 10 percent of calories per day from added sugars*
- *Consume less than 10 percent of calories per day from saturated fats*
- *Consume less than 2,300 milligrams (mg) per day of sodium*
- *If alcohol is consumed, it should be consumed in moderation—up to one drink per day for women and up to two drinks per day for men—and only by adults of legal drinking age*

In tandem with the recommendations above, Americans of all ages—children, adolescents, adults, and older adults—should meet the Physical Activity Guidelines for Americans *to help promote health and reduce the risk of chronic disease. Americans should aim to achieve and maintain a healthy body weight. The relationship between diet and physical activity contributes to calorie balance and managing body weight. As such, the* Dietary Guidelines *includes a Key Recommendation to*

- *Meet the* Physical Activity Guidelines for Americans. *(See*: http://www.health.gov/paguidelines)

According to the above *Dietary Guidelines* report, the Office of Disease Prevention and Health Promotion, the U.S. Centers for Disease Control and Prevention, and other reports (see reference list), the rates of chronic diet-related diseases have risen, due in large part to changes in lifestyle behaviors. They conclude that a history of poor eating and physical activity patterns have a cumulative effect and have contributed to significant nutrition- and physical activity-related health challenges that now face the U.S. population. According to the *Dietary Guidelines* report: "*About half of all American adults—117 million individuals—have one or more preventable chronic diseases, many of which are related to poor quality eating patterns and physical inactivity. These include cardiovascular disease, high blood pressure, type 2 diabetes, some cancers, and poor bone health. More than two-thirds of adults and nearly one-third of children and youth are overweight or obese. These high rates of overweight and obesity and chronic disease have persisted for more than two decades and come not only with increased health risks, but also at high cost. In 2008, the medical costs associated with obesity were estimated to be $147 billion. In 2012, the total estimated cost of diagnosed diabetes was $245 billion, including $176 billion in direct medical costs and $69 billion in decreased productivity.*"

In Canada, Health Canada (a branch of the Canadian government) is currently in the process of reviewing and updating its dietary guidelines in view of newer scientific evidence and, not surprisingly, appears to be reaching similar conclusions. This process will result in an update of *Canada's Food Guide*, and information about the progress of the revisions made available by the Canadian government has highlighted the key lines of evidence that will underpin the revised *Guide*. These are:

- *Association between increased intakes according to the Dietary Approaches to Stop Hypertension (DASH) pattern and decreased blood pressure or LDL cholesterol*

- *Association between increased intakes according to Mediterranean-style, Portfolio or DASH patterns and decreased LDL cholesterol or cardiovascular disease risk*

- *Association between increased intakes of foods containing dietary fibre and decreased risk of colorectal cancer*

- *Association between increased intakes of fruit and vegetables and decreased cardiovascular disease risk*

- *Association between a diet high in nuts and decreased LDL cholesterol*

- *Association between increased intakes of soy protein and decreased LDL cholesterol*

- *Association between increased intakes of red meat (beef, pork, lamb and goat) and increased risk of colorectal cancer*

- *Association between replacement of saturated fatty acids with unsaturated fatty acids and decreased LDL cholesterol or cardiovascular disease risk*

- *Association between increased intakes of sodium and increased blood pressure*

- *Association between increased intakes of added sugar (from food and/or sugar-sweetened beverages) and increased risk of obesity or type 2 diabetes*

- *Association between increased intakes of sugar-sweetened beverages and increased risk of obesity among children*

- *Association between increased intakes of sugar-containing beverages and increased risk of dental caries in children*

- *Association between replacement of saturated fatty acids with unsaturated fatty acids and decreased LDL blood cholesterol and cardiovascular disease risk*

- *Association between increased intakes of processed meat (meats processed by smoking, curing or salting, or addition of chemical preservatives) and increased risk of colorectal cancer*

Given these major health impacts of our everyday diet, it is somewhat surprising that so many people ignore these recommendations and instead focus on the trivial or nonexistent potential impacts of well-controlled food additives and residues of pesticides or hormones.

The U.S. Centers for Disease Control and Prevention (CDCP) website on chronic disease prevention and health promotion concludes that chronic diseases and conditions—such as heart disease, stroke, cancer, type 2 diabetes, obesity, and arthritis—are among the most common, costly, and preventable of all health problems. According to their statistics, seven of the top ten causes of death in 2014 were chronic diseases, with heart disease and cancer accounting for nearly 46% of all deaths. Obesity is identified as a serious health concern, with more than one-third of adults (36%), or about 84 million people, being obese during 2011-2014 (defined as body mass index [BMI] ≥30 kg/m^2). About one in six youths (17%) aged 2 to 19 years was obese. Among other important findings related to dietary factors that can be controlled is the occurrence of diabetes, which is the leading cause of kidney failure, lower-limb amputations other than those caused by injury, and new cases of blindness among adults. Four controllable key health risk behaviors that cause chronic diseases were identified by the CDCP—lack of exercise or physical activity, poor nutrition, tobacco use, and drinking too much alcohol. These practices have clearly been shown to cause much illness, suffering, and early death. Key reported facts are (https://www.cdc.gov/chronicdisease/data/index.htm):

- Six in ten adults in the U.S. have a chronic disease, many of which are caused by specific risk behaviors
- Important risk behaviors include tobacco use, poor nutrition, lack of physical activity, and excessive alcohol use
- In 2017, 46% of adults aged 18 years or older did not meet recommendations for aerobic physical activity. In addition,

76% did not meet recommendations for both aerobic and muscle-strengthening physical activity.

- In 2017, 30% of U.S. adults were obese
- In 2017, more than 35% of adults and adolescents ate fruit less than once a day, while 40% of adolescents and 19% of adults ate vegetables less than once a day.
- An estimated 34 million adults in the United States smoke cigarettes. Cigarette smoking accounts for more than 480,000 deaths each year.
- Drinking too much alcohol is responsible for 88,000 deaths each year.

Additionally:

In the United States, chronic diseases and conditions and the health risk behaviors that cause them account for most health care costs.

- Eighty-six percent of the nation's 2.7 trillion dollars annual health care expenditures are for people with chronic and mental health conditions. These costs can be reduced.
- Medical costs linked to obesity were estimated to be 147 billion dollars in 2008. Annual medical costs for people who were obese were $1,429 higher than those for people of normal weight.
- The economic cost due to smoking is estimated to be at least $300 billion a year. This cost includes nearly 170 billion dollars in direct medical care for adults.
- The economic costs of drinking too much alcohol were estimated to be 249 billion dollars, or $2.05 a drink, in 2010. Most of these costs were due to binge drinking and resulted from losses in workplace productivity, health care expenses, and crimes related to excessive drinking.

The FDA is aware of the importance of the influence of nutritional factors that are related to preventable chronic disease and has made it a priority to identify new ways to reduce the burden of chronic disease through improved nutrition. In May 2016 the FDA announced a new format for the nutrition facts label for packaged foods to reflect new scientific information, including the link between diet and chronic diseases such as obesity and heart disease. The new label is designed to make it easier to make better informed food choices. More recently, in March 2018, FDA Commissioner Gottlieb announced the FDA Nutrition Innovation Strategy, emphasizing that the FDA is committed to finding new ways to reduce the burden of chronic disease through improved nutrition by using its tools and authorities to both empower consumers with information and facilitate industry innovation toward healthy foods (https://www.fda.gov/food/food-labeling-nutrition/fda-nutrition-innovation-strategy).

Excessive levels of saturated fats, sugars, sodium, and total calories are found in many products generally considered to be healthy. This makes it critically important to use the nutritional information that is now mandated to be on the labels of all food products to avoid excessive intake of these dietary components that have been found to be associated with adverse health outcomes. The format of the currently required food labels makes it easy to identify those that contain unhealthy levels. For example, a serving of name brand chicken vegetable soup can contain approximately half of the recommended daily sodium limit, one small 6 oz. container of a leading brand of blueberry yogurt contains 38% of the recommended daily maximum sugar intake, canned fruits often contain 40-50% of the recommended daily sugar intake per serving, one slice of Swiss cheese contains 25% of the daily recommended limit of saturated fat, and one 12-inch flour tortilla can contain more than 30% of the recommended daily limit of sodium.

When making comparisons with the recommended limited intakes in the *Dietary Guidelines* it is useful to know that saturated fats contribute approximately 9 calories per gram of fat and sugars contribute about 4 calories per gram of sugar. Because the guidelines specify the daily limits of these nutrients as the percentage of total daily calories that they contribute, some arithmetic is required to calculate one's own applicable limit. To relieve consumers of the need for some of this arithmetic, the current food labels provide the percentage of the recommended daily intake of the major nutrients provided by one serving, expressed as the percent daily value (%DV) for an individual consuming a 2000 calorie per day diet. Because more active people may require a higher calorie intake and others less, some arithmetic is still necessary to adjust to your individual total calorie requirement.

Although the actual content of nutritional components specified on the label is required to be accurate, the labeling is sometimes construed to mislead the consumer. For example, one leading brand of canned black beans is prominently labeled "reduced sodium" but it actually contains almost three times the amount of sodium as another leading brand that does not carry either a "low sodium" or "reduced sodium" designation on its label. Thus, it is critical to understand the current recommended guidelines for those dietary components that should be limited, especially sodium, saturated fat, and added sugars, and to read the nutritional label to ensure that the recommended dietary guidelines are followed. The current scientific evidence shows that there are major health benefits from following these guidelines. So, read the nutrient content information on food labels and try to meet the above principal dietary recommendations! This, along with adequate exercise and sleep, is one of the most useful things one can do to ensure a long, active, and healthy life.

The extensive benefits of physical exercise have been shown in many studies and are comprehensively documented by the *2018 Physical Activity Guidelines Advisory Committee Scientific Report* to the U.S. Department of Health and Human Services (2018). Among the important conclusions of this expert scientific panel, the *Report* shows that regular physical activity provides a variety of benefits that improve health, reduce the risk of disease, and help us feel better, sleep better, and perform daily tasks more easily. Some of these benefits happen immediately. For example, a single moderate-to-vigorous physical activity can improve that night's sleep, reduce anxiety symptoms, improve cognition, reduce blood pressure, and improve insulin sensitivity on the day that it is performed. Even greater benefits are achieved with the regular performance of moderate-to-vigorous physical activity. Specific important findings of this committee are that:

- Greater amounts of moderate-to-vigorous physical activity are associated with preventing or minimizing excessive weight gain in adults, maintaining weight within a healthy range, and preventing obesity

- Higher amounts of physical activity are associated with a reduced risk of excessive increases in body weight and adiposity in children ages 3 to 17 years

- More physically active women are less likely to gain excessive weight during pregnancy. They also are less likely to develop gestational diabetes or develop postpartum depression than their less-active peers. Maternal and child health has been, appropriately, a priority in the United States for generations.

- Greater amounts of physical activity reduce the risk of dementia and improve other aspects of cognitive function

- For the first time, the 2018 *Scientific Report* demonstrates that regular physical activity provides health benefits to children as young as ages 3 to 5 years

- In addition to a reduced risk of excessive gains in body weight and adiposity, regular physical activity improves bone health in this young age group

- For older adults, strong evidence demonstrates a reduced risk of falls and fall-related injuries

- The 2008 Committee concluded that regular moderate-to-vigorous physical activity reduced the risk of breast and colon cancer. The 2018 Committee expanded that list to include a reduced risk for cancers of the bladder, endometrium, esophagus, kidney, lung, and stomach.

- A large portion of the general population already has a chronic disease or condition. For many of these individuals, regular physical activity can reduce the risk of developing a new chronic condition, reduce the risk of progression of the condition they already have, and improve their quality of life and physical function. The conditions examined by the Committee included some of the most prevalent, including osteoarthritis, hypertension, and type 2 diabetes.

Importantly, physical exercise may be one of the most effective ways to improve cognitive loss in people with "mild cognitive impairment", which is often a precursor to full-blown Alzheimer's disease. For example, a study by J. Carson Smith and colleagues at the University of Maryland in collaboration with other scientists (Smith *et al.*, 2013) has shown that regular, moderate exercise can improve memory and cognitive function in older adults with mild cognitive impairment who are at risk for Alzheimer's disease. No drugs are currently available that can achieve comparable results. Given the extent of cognitive impairment in the elderly and the impact of this condition on their lives and their loved ones, this is a very important finding.

The relationship between cancer risk and diet has been the subject of intensive research for more than 50 years, since differences in certain cancers in different geographical areas were found to be correlated with dietary practices. In the late 1970s the famous British epidemiologists Sir Richard Doll and Sir Richard Peto were commissioned by the U.S. Congress Office of Technology Assessment to produce a report on the percentages of cancers that could be attributed to avoidable causes. This report was published in 1981 (Doll and Peto, 1981), and has since been a benchmark against which recent reviews have compared estimates of cancer risk based on additional scientific information that has become available since that time (*e.g.*, Willett, 1995; Blot and Tarone, 2015). Current estimates are that about 20-32% of cancer could be avoided by dietary changes. These estimates depend in part on differences in cancer rates among areas with different dietary composition, but the specific dietary factors responsible for the observed differences have not been clearly differentiated. Nonetheless, saturated fat and red meat consumption are strongly correlated with colon cancer rates and intake of fresh fruits and vegetables in conjunction with a low saturated fat diet appears to be protective, although recent studies suggest that the effect on many cancers may be more modest than original estimates suggested.

Given the many health benefits of adequate exercise and physical activity, it is disappointing that the 2010-2015 *Dietary Guidelines* report states that based on 2013 data only approximately 20% of U.S. adults meet the physical activity guidelines of the 2008 physical activities advisory committee, and that the percentages are even less in age groups over 55. The scientific evidence is overwhelming that the combination of more active physical exercise and improved diet has the potential for major health improvements and disease prevention.

Another important factor is sleep. Sleep deficiency has been associated with modifications in immune function, mood, learning ability, cognitive function, memory, glucose tolerance and type 2 diabetes risks, and appetite and body weight maintenance. The scientific literature documenting these effects is complex and more difficult to access because there are not authoritative expert reviews mandated and supported by the government, as is the case with the effects of diet and exercise. The interested reader may consult the Wikipedia articles on sleep and sleep deprivation that provide references for further reading on effects of inadequate sleep and the benefits of getting sufficient sleep (*e.g.*, see https://en.wikipedia.org/wiki/Sleep_deprivation; https://en.wikipedia.org/wiki/Effects_of_sleep_deprivation_on_cognitive_performance). Among these effects are modification of leptin and ghrelin levels, hormones that control appetite and can lead to hunger and weight gain—leading to the attendant negative health effects of obesity. Such endocrine alterations have been found to occur even after a single night of sleep restriction.

In contrast to the well-documented impact of the above major health factors, there are no well-accepted data showing that food additives and pesticide residues that conform to current regulatory standards have any significant adverse human health impact.

Chapter 13

Recommendations for Consumers— and for Legislators and Regulatory Authorities

The information in the preceding chapters is intended to provide a perspective that will help consumers make better choices of consumable products and to ask better questions of doctors, dieticians, pharmacists, and other health care professionals. It is also intended to call the attention of regulatory professionals and legislators to the need to address the current discrepancies in safety assurance among the different types of products that have been discussed. Hopefully it will be a motivation to modify existing safety regulations, and where necessary the controlling legislation, to provide more uniformity across product classes. Some personal suggestions to consumers and to the professionals responsible for the regulatory framework that determines the degree of safety of our food, drug, and dietary supplement products follow.

For Consumers

Although it isn't possible to offer detailed information about specific products, some general recommendations can be made with regard to the issues that have been discussed.

First, don't be misled by advertising that suggests that "natural" and "organic" products are necessarily preferred over conventional products that have been produced with the use of pesticides or additives. The use of pesticides and food additives increases crop yields, reduces plant stress from insect or microbial attack, stabilizes products, prevents harmful degradation, and improves taste and sensory appeal. When considering whether the additional cost of an organic food is a good investment, remember that all plants contain a vast array of naturally occurring chemicals that have evolved to protect the plant from predation and plant diseases and to interact in other ways with organisms in the plant's environment. Some of these secondary metabolites serve the same functions and have biological properties similar to the synthetic pesticides, pest deterrents, and additives that are used in conventional food production. In general, those endogenous chemicals have not been systematically studied in the laboratory to determine their health effects. Compared with conventionally produced foods, those endogenous chemicals with the greatest biological activity may be elevated in organic products because of breeding for pest resistance or stress-induced synthesis due to insect or microbial attack that may occur in the absence of the use of pesticidal agents. My own conviction is that residues of commercially used pesticides and permitted levels of food additives are well-studied, well-controlled, and are not a significant health concern. In fact, their use makes available lower-cost healthy foods produced under conditions less stressful to the crops on which they are used. Keeping these issues in mind:

- Educate yourself and maintain a reasonable perspective about relative benefits and risks, keeping in mind the examples presented in previous chapters. Be aware of the laws governing the marketing and sales of dietary and pharmaceutical products, and the meaning of labeling statements. Act on facts rather than distorted perceptions of risk engendered by mistaken assumptions that natural products are necessarily safer than those developed by humans or that plants exist mainly for the benefit of humans.

- Be aware that those products that are most thoroughly studied will essentially always have some documented reports of health effects at high exposure levels because it is necessary to test exposures up to a level that produces an adverse effect in order to establish a safe allowable level that won't produce that effect under actual conditions of use. The levels permitted in foods are set using very conservative safety margins that allow for uncertainties in data extrapolation, individual sensitivities, and other factors. Products that have not been thoroughly studied will necessarily lack comprehensive information about potential adverse health effects and adequate safety margins will therefore not have been established. Those who sell inadequately tested products may attempt to mislead you into believing that the more thoroughly tested product has numerous "toxic effects" by citing the reports of studies conducted to determine safety margins that assure safety. The more thoroughly tested product is almost certainly the safer and thorough testing of the other would almost always result in reports of toxicities at high doses.

- Recognize that the health risk of any chemical is intrinsically linked to the level of exposure and that almost all chemicals exhibit toxicity at some level of exposure. Balance your judgments based on the knowledge of how thoroughly each class of product has been evaluated and whether reports of adverse effects occur at exposures that are near those that occur during the use of the product.

- Do not be misled by qualitative statements about potential health effects based on effects that have been demonstrated at excessively high exposures that are not relevant to actual usage conditions. The risk of health effects from chemical exposures is meaningful only when the extent and level of exposure is known in the context of exposure-response characteristics of the chemical. For example, an appropriate amount of vitamin A is essential for good health and nutrition but an excessive amount is toxic and causes liver damage—therefore the statement that "consuming vitamin A is essential for good health" and the alternative statement that "consuming vitamin A can kill you" are equally true. Don't be taken in by statements made out of context.

- Eat a normal nutritionally balanced diet with a variety of fruits and vegetables and a balanced content of major nutrients, exercise regularly, and get plenty of sleep. Refer to the U.S. *Dietary Guidelines* discussed in the previous chapter and modify your diet to conform to those recommendations. While organic produce is probably not a major health risk, conventionally grown produce is at least as safe and possibly safer and is far less costly. Pesticides used in commercial food production have been extensively evaluated and residues are controlled to levels that are of negligible health risk; organic produce that has been selected for "natural" disease resistance has probably not been subjected to comprehensive safety studies and the factors responsible for their disease resistance are generally not well-studied.

- If your food budget is restricted, remember that the health benefits of a well-balanced diet high in fresh vegetables and fruits are well-documented and do not choose expensive organic and preservative-free products if their expense causes you to limit your intake of wholesome fresh fruits and vegetables.

- Don't be misguided by the general belief that the "organic" label means that a product is better. Choose fruits and vegetables of high quality because plants produce defensive chemicals and secondary metabolites when subjected to stress and damage and are also subject to microbial and fungal infection when stressed or damaged. These factors likely are responsible for more risk than are well-studied pesticide residues. Pesticide use in the United States is rigorously controlled and the benefits of consuming a diet rich in fruits and vegetables far outweigh the risk of an adverse health effect from pesticide residues. If you can afford it and wish to pay more for a pesticide-free organic product, that is probably not a great risk from a safety point of view as long as the product is of high quality and is not stressed or damaged.

- Choose intelligently, recognizing the liabilities of products not evaluated by the FDA. Look for the telltale disclaimer: "*These statements have not been evaluated by the U.S. Food and Drug Administration*". This indicates that this product is regulated under the DSHEA and that the FDA has probably not reviewed either the product safety or the accuracy of the health claims made for the product. Products with this labeling may be sold with minimal or no safety testing.

- Be aware that adulteration of botanical supplements regulated under the DSHEA is widespread and that the FDA has limited resources to identify adulteration and to enforce control over these products.

- Avoid "quick fixes" and "miracle products", such as weight loss products, sexual activity enhancers, stimulant products (energy enhancers), etc., that have not been evaluated in double-blind trials for safety and efficacy. Recognize that illegal spiking of botanical supplements with prescription drugs or unapproved biologically active chemicals is rampant, especially in the cases of products marketed for enhancement of sexual enhancement, weight loss, or improvement of athletic performance. Many of these adulterated products are dangerous and may cause serious injury or even death.

- If you choose to purchase organic products, be aware of the differences between the labeling statements, *e.g.* "100% organic", "organic", and listings of specific organic ingredients.

- Recognize that organic products have not been demonstrated to be nutritionally superior to, or safer than, conventional food products. Although low-level residues of certain pesticides and food additives will be absent from such products, such chemicals have generally been well-studied and controlled to levels that don't present a significant health risk. Organic products may have been selected for disease resistance and thereby contain uncharacterized natural constituents with unknown health effects.

- Paying a premium to avoid tiny amounts of well-studied food additives, such as phenolic antioxidant food additives, while also paying a premium to purchase "natural" food products that contain similar chemicals (such as açaí berries that have higher levels of similar phenolic antioxidants) but have not been subjected to comprehensive safety studies does not make sense.

- Before selecting products labeled "not tested in animals", be aware that many important health effects cannot be detected unless animal testing is conducted. Also, such labeling on cosmetic products is often deceptive because the final product may not have been tested in animals but the active ingredients in the product may have been tested. Hopefully better *in vitro* test systems and computer prediction models will become available in the future and will allow less animal testing. Indeed, modern methods have already been implemented that have achieved significant decreases in animal testing, but there is near-unanimous consensus among scientists involved in safety testing that it is not possible at the present time to assure safety without some animal (or human) testing.

For Regulatory Agencies and Legislators

Regulatory agencies generally focus available resources on the regulation of those products for which strict regulatory mandates are already in place and for which the product sponsor or marketer is required to provide rigorous scientific proof of the product's safety and efficacy prior to approval for sale. When existing regulations and laws do not explicitly define safety testing requirements, and when the burden to prove harm or undue risk of harm is on the regulatory agency rather than on the Sponsor, fewer resources are generally allocated to the safety evaluation of such products. Given the extremely high cost of product safety and efficacy testing and the length of time necessary to complete such testing this is understandable, but, unfortunately, this tendency means that even if the product usage is potentially more dangerous it is often less well studied. Also, responsibility for products is often divided across multiple agencies, and this often leads to disparate risk evaluation standards. Nonetheless, government regulatory bodies have a public and moral responsibility to evaluate and act upon those products under their jurisdiction that are most likely to present the greatest health risks, even when the complexity of the current laws and regulations limit the ability to redirect resources.

Some of the key issues that need to be addressed with regard to the safety assurance of botanical supplements and organic foods are:

1. It is time to consider reframing the current health and safety laws related to foods, drugs, dietary supplements, cosmetics, and agricultural products into a simplified but comprehensive law that assures uniform safety standards across these product classes, and to assure that research and testing focus on the products that present the highest health risks.

2. More rigorous identity and purity standards for botanical products with variable and complex chemical compositions that depend not only on the plant species but also on the genetics of the specific cultivar, growing conditions, disease stressors, and other factors should be implemented.

3. The extensive use of multiple pharmaceuticals in combination with botanical supplements by an aging population increases the need for better protection against drug interactions.

4. Scientific principles dictate that an equal level of safety assurance should be required for all substances intentionally ingested by the public, yet controlled safety studies of marketed botanicals are often lacking. Steps that can be taken, within existing laws, to bring safety standards for botanical products into line with those for pharmaceuticals, foods, and food additives need to be defined.

A focus on the above issues by the regulatory and legislative communities is needed. Some specific recommendations follow:

- Educational programs are needed that increase public understanding of hazard identification, risk assessment, and the scientific evidence upon which both are based. Programs should include information for the general adult public and also elementary level education that enhances an understanding of:

  1) the scientific method, its uncertainties, and the need for independent confirmation of scientific hypotheses and theories

2) the general principles of risk assessment and the dependence of risk on the extent of exposure to hazards

3) the need for experimental evidence that tests hypotheses from multiple perspectives

4) the fact that no evidence of risk is *not* evidence of no risk unless appropriate safety studies have been carried out

- Repeal DSHEA and bring the regulation of botanical supplements under a framework similar to that under which food additives, pesticide residues, and pharmaceutical products are regulated

- Pass a new comprehensive law that simplifies the current regulatory structure and reframes safety regulations so that all products within similar classes are regulated to comparable standards

- Combine those agency segments with the responsibility to regulate food and dietary supplement products into a single food agency with the responsibility to regulate all food and dietary supplement products, including food additives and pesticide residues in food, under a single set of regulatory testing and evaluation standards. Merging this responsibility would allow oversight by a consolidated intellectual resource of health professionals who could apply consistent standards across all ingested products (foods, nutritional supplements, drinking water, and food additives, including contaminants and residues therein). It would also likely be more cost-effective than the current segmented system.

- Therapeutic drugs, botanical health supplements, dietary supplements (including vitamins and minerals) all serve the purpose of improving health and reducing the risks associated with diseases, and should be regulated under a single set of testing standards that ensure efficacy, safety, and product quality (uniformity of manufacturing, confirmation of identity, lack of impurities, etc.). Regulatory authority for both drugs and dietary supplements that make structure-function and health claims should be under the same agency center.

- Cosmetic products should be subject to premarket testing requirements that assure their safety and the accuracy of health and cosmetic claims. Testing requirements should include the most relevant systems available, reducing animal testing in cases that do not compromise safety assurance. Claims that the product has not been tested in animals should not be permitted when ingredients that comprise the product have been tested in animals.

- More resources should be focused on food products. There is a disparity between the regulation of food, which we consume in large quantities every day, and food additives and pesticides, to which we have much lower and/or more intermittent exposures. Foods constitute our greatest daily exposure to exogenous chemicals and yet are among the least rigorously evaluated of our exposures. This is due to the assumption that food must be safe because it is necessary for our survival and we have been consuming it for a long time.

- Provide a more uniform approach to research and regulation related to dietary constituents that influence disease. Studies have shown that diet is a major determinant of cardiovascular disease, diseases related to metabolic or immunological disorders, and overall cancer rates. Carcinogenic substances are known to occur in foods but safety regulations treat naturally occurring and added substances differently. Agents that have been shown to cause cancer are not allowed to be added to foods at any level, but naturally occurring carcinogenic substances are not regulated unless the FDA can provide scientific evidence that in fact they are causing harm. Further, the potential of the many thousands of chemical constituents of foods have not been systematically screened to determine which may have the potential to induce or promote cancer. This includes many secondary metabolites in foods that are known to cause mutations, a property associated with cancer induction. Modern screening methods that allow identification of mutagenic and other cancer-related properties can now efficiently identify agents with potential cancer-causing properties and these could be applied to systematic studies. In fact, such studies can now in some cases be conducted directly in humans under conditions of controlled dietary exposures.

- Form a consortium of experts from government, academic, non-government, and private organizations to develop recommendations for improved safety evaluation and regulation of botanical products, especially botanical supplements. This is a special need due to the chemical complexity of plant-derived products, which generally contain many biologically active endogenous chemicals that vary with specific genetic lines, in response to growth conditions and environmental stress, location within parts of the plant, etc. A group of interdisciplinary scientific experts with expertise in plant chemistry, safety evaluation, and the existing regulatory structure could bring a fresh perspective and innovative recommendations for modified regulatory and legislative approaches to improve identity and safety standards for these products.

- Focus on the safety of older products. In all classes, older products have been allowed to remain on the market without updating safety testing to current standards. For example, older approved drugs are rarely studied because the burden of proof following approval shifts to the FDA. Foods and food additives in use prior to 1958 are "grandfathered" and assumed to be safe (*i.e.*, are GRAS, or generally recognized as safe). Supplements in use before the 1994 DSHEA law are exempted from the requirement to file a New Dietary Ingredient Notification to the FDA and need not be tested by the Sponsor prior to sale, etc. Thus, these older products are not held to the same safety standards as are new products. Even when safety issues are identified with these older products, they are often allowed to remain on the market because regulatory action would require demonstration of health risk by the regulatory agency and the resources to perform conclusive studies are often not available to the responsible regulatory agency.

- Increase federally funded grants to study products currently on the market that have not been tested to current standards, including foods, dietary supplements, food additives classified as GRAS, and drugs approved prior to implementation of current testing standards. If grant-funded research identifies potential risks, then regulations could be applied or further studies undertaken to determine the magnitude of potential health risks. This would allow universities and non-governmental scientific institutions to undertake studies that are beyond the capacity of the government to implement.

- Regulations should be implemented that require consistent scientific evidence that supports labeling claims, with a specified timeline for bringing products already on the market into compliance with consistent evidential standards, to ensure:

  - That all health claims are supported by data from one or more controlled studies and have been reviewed and approved by the consolidated regulatory agency prior to sale of the product

- That products used and labeled to treat or prevent a disease or abnormal condition, or to sustain or improve general health or the health of a specific organ or organ system, have been tested and proven to be both safe and effective under the conditions of use in accord with the standards already in place for pharmaceutical drugs.

- Establish a uniform adverse event reporting system that extends and modifies the current FDA adverse event reporting system. This system should have two components: 1) the spontaneous event reporting system that already exists, to establish a record of cases in which an adverse event appears to be linked to exposure to a particular product, and 2) defined prospective population surveys where the number of individuals exposed and at risk, the level of exposure, and the frequency of adverse events are determined in order to establish quantitative estimates of potential risk. Consideration could be given to linking existing databases such as patient databases from large health care organizations, data from the nHANES nutrition survey, and other sources by obtaining the consent of surveyed individuals. On a broader scale, a national medical records system through which the medical records of all citizens could be accessed *via* the internet is badly needed. If this were established it could be linked to adverse event reporting systems. This would dramatically decrease the cost and increase the sensitivity of associative epidemiology studies, as well as reducing medical care costs by eliminating the need for unnecessary repetition of expensive medical tests when individuals move, are away from home, or change doctors. Current computer technology has the capability to identify significant associations long before a human would notice the same correlations. As part of such a program, implement a higher level of interaction with foreign countries that have nationalized health care systems.

Cooperative studies among countries could greatly increase the efficiency of resource utilization.

- Perform a physician survey to assess needed areas of improvement related to reporting of adverse events. Based on informal discussions with general practitioners, it appears that very few physicians file reports using the current prescription drug adverse event reporting system, and that even those that do often don't report events when they feel unsure of an association or when they observe events that they feel must already be known. A plan that improves utilization of the reporting systems may be needed, including incentives that encourage busy health care practitioners to participate more fully.

- There should be government-wide review of discrepant standards of risk control, with the objective of recommending a relatively uniform standard that provides a consistent level of protection for different types of products. Such a standard would need to recognize that adjustments for benefit *vs.* risk must be taken into account. For example, the benefit of curing, preventing, or alleviating a serious disease justifies acceptance of greater risks for effective drug products. Likewise, it may not be possible to lower the carcinogenic risk contributed by all food products to a level as low as that to which a new food additive may be regulated. Thus, while it is not feasible or desirable to control exposure of every agent to identical levels of health risk, every effort should be made to ensure that highly discrepant standards are identified and eliminated.

Closing Comments

It is hoped that the information and examples presented will lead to more informed and better choices by consumers, and that they will also stimulate a re-assessment of current food, agricultural, pharmaceutical, and cosmetic safety laws and regulations. Hopefully, educators will take note of the importance of the science of risk-benefit analysis and management, its dependence on scientific data generated using the scientific method of experimentation to evaluate and "prove"/disprove cause and effect relationships in our everyday lives, and will place more emphasis on these subjects at an early stage of education. Consumers can reflect on the principles and recommendations presented herein, focus on sensible choices that optimize health-related product selections, and recognize misleading product claims that confuse the relative benefits and risks of different products. Most importantly, implementation of a simplified and more uniform set of safety regulations for the products discussed would assure more comparable levels of safety assurance across product classes and lead to more efficient application and enforcement of consumer health and safety regulations, thereby providing a major health benefit to the general population.

Acknowledgments

I am indebted to my wife Judith, a professional toxicologist as well as an avid reader, for her many helpful suggestions during the preparation of this book—and for tolerating the many hours I spent working on it. Her knowledge of the subject matter as a technical professional, combined with her experience as a reader of a wide range of writing styles of popular books, give her a unique perspective that was most helpful to me in my endeavor to address both a public and regulatory professional audience. My daughter, Jennifer MacGregor, M.D., was also most helpful and her experience in writing technical medical articles for the public was a great asset to me.

I also thank my many additional colleagues and friends, too numerous to list here, who provided useful comments on specific aspects of this work. I especially want to thank Jeanette Turansky and Paula Himowitz for their feedback on my early drafts, which helped guide me toward this final product. Deborah Perdue of Illumination Graphics provided exceptional professional, artistic, and timely assistance in the production of the cover and setup of the interior design.

References and Further Reading

Chapter 1: Introduction

Bailey RL, Gahche JJ, Lentino CV, Dwyer JT, Engel JS, Thomas PR, Betz JM, Sempos CT, Picciano MF (2011) Dietary supplement use in the United States, 2003-2006. Journal of Nutrition 141(2): 261-266.

Consumer Reports, The Cost of Organic Food, March 19, 2015. www.consumerreports.org/cro/news/2015/03/cost-of-organic-food/index.htm (accessed 6/5/2019)

Navarro VJ, Barnhart H, Bonkovsky HL, Davern T, Fontana RJ, Grant L, *et al.* (2014) Liver injury from herbals and dietary supplements in the U.S. Drug-Induced Liver Injury Network. Hepatology 60: 1399-1408.

Smith T, Kawa K, Eckl V, Morton C, Stredney R (2018) Sales of herbal dietary supplements in U.S. increased 8.5% in 2017, topping $8 billion. HerbalGram. 119: 62-71. (http://cms.herbalgram.org/herbalgram/issue119/hg119-herbmktrpt.html) (Accessed 6/5/2019)

U.S. Department of Agriculture, Economic Research Service, Tables of Organic Prices, Updated March 7, 2016. http://ers.usda.gov/data-products/organic-prices.aspx (Accessed 6/5/2019)

U.S. Food and Drug Administration (2019) Statement from FDA Commissioner Scott Gottlieb, M.D., on the agency's new efforts to strengthen regulation of dietary supplements by modernizing and reforming FDA's oversight, February 11, 2019 (www.fda.gov/news-events/press-announcements/statement-fda-commissioner-scott-gottlieb-md-agencys-new-efforts-strengthen-regulation-dietary) (accessed 6/5/2019)

Chapter 2: Plants Are Not Benign

Balandrin MF, Klocke JA, Wurtele ES, Bollinger WH (1985) Natural plant chemicals: sources of industrial and medicinal materials. Science 228: 1154-1160.

Bennett RM, Wallsgrove RM (1994) Tansley Review No. 72: Secondary metabolites in plant defence. New Phytologist 127: 647-633. (http://onlinelibrary.wiley.com/doi/10.1111/j.1469-8137.1994.tb02968.x/pdf) (Accessed 6/5/2019)

Clark AM (1982) Endogenous mutagens in green plants, in "Environmental Mutagenesis, Carcinogenesis, and Plant Biology", Vol I, ed. Klekowski EJ, Jr., Praeger Scientific, Greenwood Publishing Group, Inc., Westport, CT, pp. 97-132.

Cosmetic Ingredient Review Expert Panel (2004) Final report of the amended safety assessment of Dioscorea Villosa (Wild Yam) root extract. Int. J. Toxicol. 23: Suppl. 2: 49-54.

Diamond, Jared (1999) *Guns, Germs and Steel: The fates of human societies*, W.W. Norton & Co., Inc., 500 5th Avenue, New York, NY 10110.

Dodds PN, Rathjen JP (2010) Plant immunity: towards an integrated view of plant-pathogen interactions. Nature Reviews-Genetics 11: 539-548.

Farmer EE, Ryan CA (1990) Interplant communication: Airborne methyl jasmonate induces synthesis of proteinase inhibitors in plant leaves, Proc. Natl. Acad. Sci. USA 87: 7713-7716.

Göggelmann W, Schimmer O (1986) Mutagenic activity of phytotherapeutical drugs, in *Genetic Toxicology of the Diet*, ed. Kundsen I, Prog. Clin. Biol. Res., vol 206, Alan R. Liss, New York, pp. 63-72.

Kikuta Y, Ueda H, Nakayama K, Katsuda Y, Ozawa R, Takabayashi J, Hatanaka A, Matsuda K (2011) Specific regulation of pyrethrin biosynthesis in *Chrysanthemum cinerariaefolium* by a blend of volatiles emitted from artificially damaged conspecific plants. Plant Cell Physiol. 52(3): 588-96.

Knudsen I (1986) *Genetic Toxicology of the Diet*, Prog. Clin. Biol. Res., vol 206, Alan R. Liss, New York, 351 pp.

Laursen T, Borch J, Knudsen C, Bevishi K, Torta F, *et al.* (2016) Characterization of a dynamic metabolon producing the defense compound dhurrin in sorghum. Science 354: 890-893.

Mazid M, Khan TA, Mohammad F (2011) Role of secondary metabolites in defense mechanisms of plants. Biology and Medicine 3: 232-249.

Pennisi E (2015) How crop-killing witchweed senses its victims. Science 350: 146-147.

Pollan M (2013) The Intelligent Plant. The New Yorker, December 23 & 30, 2013 Issue (www.newyorker.com/magazine/2013/12/23/the-intelligent-plant) (Accessed 6/5/2019)

Shang Y, Ma Y, Zhou Y, Zhang H, Duan L, Chen H, Zeng J, Zhou Q, Wang S, Gu W, Liu M, Ren J, Gu X, Zhang S, Wang Y, Yasukawa K, Bouwmeester HJ, Qi X, Zhang Z, Lucas WJ, Huang S (2014) Biosynthesis, regulation, and domestication of bitterness in cucumber. Science 346: 1084-1088.

Stokstad E (2016) How the Venus flytrap acquired its taste for meat. Science 352: 756.

Tamura G, Gold C, Ferro-Luzzi A, Ames BN (1980) Fecalase: A model for activation of dietary glycosides to mutagens by intestinal flora. Proc. Natl. Acad. Sci. USA 77: 4961-4965.

Theis N, Lerdau M (2003) The evolution of function in plant secondary metabolites. Int. Journal of Plant Sci. 164 (3 Suppl.): S93-S102.

van der Hoeven JC, Lagerweij WJ, Bruggeman IM, Voragen FG, Koeman JH (1983) Mutagenicity of extracts of some vegetables commonly consumed in the Netherlands. J. Agricultural and Food Chemistry 31: 1020-1026.

Wasternack C, Feussner I. The Oxylipin Pathways: Biochemistry and Function, Annual Review of Plant Biology, 69: 363-386, April 2018. (https://www.annualreviews.org/doi/10.1146/annurev-arplant-042817-040440) (Accessed 6/5/2019)

Wink, M. (editor) (1999) Functions of Plant Secondary Metabolites and their Exploitation in Biotechnology, CRC Press (US and Canada) and Sheffield Academic Press (England), 362 pp.

Yahiaoui R, Guechi A, Lukasova E, Girre L (1994) Mutagenic and membranal effect of a phytotoxic molecule isolated from olive trees parasitized by the fungus *Cycloconium oleaginium* Cast. Mycopathologia 126: 121-129.

Chapter 3: Toxic Effects and Their Causes Can Be Hard to Identify

Abourashad EA, El-Alfy AT, Khan IA, Walker L (2003) *Ephedra* in perspective—a current review. Phytother. Research 17(7): 703-712.

Bamias G and Boletis J (2008) Balkan nephropathy: evolution of our knowledge. Am. J. Kidney Dis. 52: 606-616.

Beutler E (2008) Glucose-6-phosphate dehydrogenase deficiency: a historical perspective. Blood 111(1): 16-24.

Centers for Disease Control and Prevention, Anticholinergic poisoning associated with an herbal tea—New York City, 1994, March 1995, Morbidity and Mortality Weekly Report, 44(11): 193-195. March 24, 1995.

Centers for Disease Control and Prevention, Cardiac valvulopathy associated with exposure to fenfluramine or dexfenfluramine: U.S. Department of Health and Human Services Interim Public Health Recommendations, November 1997, Morbidity and Mortality Weekly Report, 46(45) 1061-1066, November 14, 1997.

Connolly HM, Crary JL, McGoon MD, Hensrud DD, Edwards BS, Edwards WD, Schaff HV (1997) Valvular heart disease associated with fenfluramine-phentermine. New Eng. J. Med. 337: 581-588.

Cosyns JP (2003) Aristolochic acid and "Chinese herbs nephropathy": a review of the evidence to date. Drug Safety 26: 33-48.

Davis SA, Feldman SR, Taylor SL (2014) Use of St. John's wort in potentially dangerous combinations. J. Altern. Complement. Med. 20(7): 578-579.

Debelle FD, *et al.* (2008) Aristolochic acid nephropathy: a worldwide problem. Kidney Int. 74(2): 158-69.

Grollman AP, *et al.* (2007) Aristolochic acid and the etiology of endemic (Balkan) nephropathy. Proc. Natl. Acad. Science (USA) 104: 12129-12134.

Gurley BJ (2012) Pharmacokinetic herb-drug interactions (part 1): origins, mechanisms, and the impact of botanical dietary supplements. Planta Med. 78(13): 1478-1489.

Gurley BJ, Fifer EK, Gardner Z (2012a) Pharmacokinetic herb-drug interactions (part 2): drug interactions involving popular botanical dietary supplements and their clinical relevance. Planta Med. 78(13):1490-1514.

Gurley BJ, Swain A, Hubbard MA, Williams DK, Barone G, Hartsfield F, Tong Y, Carrier DJ, Cheboyina S, Battu SK (2008) Clinical assessment of CYP2D6-mediated herb-drug interactions in humans: effects of milk thistle, black cohosh, goldenseal, kava kava, St. John's wort, and Echinacea. Molecular Nutrition & Food Research 52(7): 755-763.

Jelaković B, *et al.* (2011) Aristolactam-DNA adducts are a biomarker of environmental exposure to aristolochic acid. Kidney Int. 9 Nov 2011; doi10.1038/ki.2011.37 .

Krishna YR, Mittal V, Fiel MI Schiano T (2011) Acute liver failure caused by 'fat burners' and dietary supplements: A case report and literature review, Canadian Journal of Gastroenterology 25(3): 157-160.

Kurzbaum A, Safori G, Monir M, Simsolo C (2008) Anticholinergic syndrome in response to lupin seed toxicity. Israeli Journal of Emergency Medicine 8(2): 20-22.

NIH (2013) *Ephedra*, National Center for Complementary and Integrative Health, National Institutes of Health. (https://nccih.nih.gov/health/ephedra) (Accessed 2/15/2019)

Navarro VJ, Barnhart H, Bonkovsky HL, Davern T, Fontana RJ, Grant L, *et al.* (2014) Liver injury from herbals and dietary supplements in the U.S. Drug-Induced Liver Injury Network. Hepatology 60: 1399-1408.

Navarro V, Khan I, Björnsson, Sceff LB, Serrano J, Hoofnagle JH (2016) Liver injury from herbal and dietary supplements, Hepatology, Epub ahead of print, Nov 17, 2016, doi:10.1002/hep.28813.

Nortier JL, *et al.* (2000) Urothelial carcinoma associated with the use of a Chinese herb (*Aristolochia fangchi*). The New England Journal of Medicine 342: 1686-1692.

Pulla P (2015) A child-killing toxin emerges from the shadows. Science 348: 15-16.

Shrivastava A, Padmini S, Kumar A, *et al.*, (2015) Outbreaks of unexplained neurologic illness – Muzaffarpur, India, 2013-2014. Centers for Disease Control and Prevention, Morbidity and Mortality Weekly Report 64(03): 49-53, January 30, 2015.

Spencer PS, Palmer VS, Mazumdar R (2015) Probable toxic cause for suspected lychee-linked viral encephalitis. Emerging Infectious Diseases 21: 904-905. (http://dx.doi.org/10.3201/eid2105.141650)

Stefanovic V, Radovanovic Z (2008) Balkan endemic nephropathy and associated urothelial cancer. Nat. Clin. Pract. Urology 5: 105-112.

Stiborová M, *et al.* (1999) Aristolactam Ia metabolite of aristolochic acid I upon activation forms an adduct found in DNA of patients with Chinese herbs nephropathy. Exp. Toxicol. Pathol. 51: 421-427.

Tanchev Y, Evstatiev Z, Dorossiev D, Pencheva J, Tzvetkova G. (1956) Studies on the nephritides in the District of Vratza. *Savremena Medicina* 7: 14–29. (Bulgarian).

Tatu CA, *et al.* (1998) The etiology of Balkan Endemic Nephropathy: Still more questions than answers. Environ. Health Perspectives 106: 689-700.

U.S. Food and Drug Administration (2004) Final rule declaring dietary supplements containing ephedrine alkaloids adulterated because they present an unreasonable risk. *Federal Register.* 69(28): 6788–6854.

U.S. Food and Drug Administration, Avoiding Drug Interactions, consumer website, (www.fda.gov/ForConsumers/ConsumerUpdates/ucm096386.htm) (accessed 6/5/2019)

Vanherwegham JL, *et al.* (1993) Rapidly progressive interstitial renal fibrosis in young women: Association with slimming regimen including Chinese herbs. Lancet 341: 387-391.

Wikipedia (2016) Ephedra. (http://en.wikipedia.org/wiki/Ephedra) (accessed 6/5/2019).

Wikipedia (2016a) Glucose-6-phosphate dehydrogenase deficiency. (https:// en.wikipedia.org/wiki/Glucose-6-phosphate dehydrogenase deficiency) (accessed 6/4/2019)

Chapter 4: The Regulatory Framework

Pacheco-Palencia L, Duncan CE, Talcott ST (2009) Phytochemical composition and thermal stability of two commercial Açaí species, *Euterpe oleracea* and *Euterpe precatoria.* Food Chemistry 115: 1199-1205.

U.S. Code of Federal Regulations (2017) Title 21—Food and Drugs, Subchapter B—Food for Human Consumption, Part 172—Food Additives Permitted for Direct Addition to Food for Human Consumption, Subpart B—Food Preservatives, Sec. 172.115 BHT (21CFR172.115).

Chapter 5: The Natural Mistake

Arnon SS, Schechter R, Inglesby TV, Henderson DA, Bartlett JG, Ascher MS, Eitzen E, Fine AD, Hauer J, Layton M, Lillibridge S, Osterholm MT, O'Toole

T, Parker G, Perl TM, Russell PK, Swerdlow DL, Tonat K; Working Group on Civilian Biodefense (2001) Botulinum toxin as a biological weapon: medical and public health management. J. American Medical Assn. 285(8): 1059-1070. Erratum in JAMA 2001 Apr 25, 285(16): 2081.

Baldini EH (2017) Women and lung cancer, UpToDate (www.uptodate.com/contents/women-and-lung-cancer (Accessed 6/5/2019)

Boyles S (2017) WHO: Global smoking deaths to hit 8 million annually by 2030, MedPage Today, January 11, 2017.

CDC (2006) History of the Surgeon General's Reports on Smoking and Health, https://www.cdc.gov/tobacco/data_statistics/sgr/history/index.htm (Accessed 6/5/2019)

Egleston BL, Meireles SI, Flieder DB, Clapper ML (2009) Population-based Trends in Lung Cancer Incidence in Women. Semin. Oncology 36(6): 506-515. (www.ncbi.nlm.nih.gov/pmc/articles/PMC2846780/) (Accessed 6/5/2019)

Sugimura T (1982) Mutagens, carcinogens, and tumor promoters in our daily food. Cancer 49: 1970-1984.

U.S. Department of Health and Human Services (2014) The Health Consequences of Smoking: 50 Years of Progress. A Report of the Surgeon General, Atlanta, GA: U.S. Department of Health and Human Services, Centers for Disease Control and Prevention, National Center for Chronic Disease Prevention and Health Promotion, Office on Smoking and Health, 2014.
(https://www.ncbi.nlm.nih.gov/books/NBK179276/pdf/Bookshelf_NBK179276.pdf) (Accessed 6/5/2019)

U.S. Food and Drug Administration (2018) Dietary Supplements Guidance Documents & Regulatory Information, https://www.fda.gov/food/guidance-documents-regulatory-information-topic-food-and-dietary-supplements/dietary-supplements-guidance-documents-regulatory-information#qhc (accessed 6/5/2019)

U.S. Food and Drug Administration (2019) New Dietary Ingredients (NDI) Notification Process, https://www.fda.gov/food/dietary-supplements/new-dietary-ingredients-ndi-notification-process (accessed 6/5/2019)

Wikipedia (2017) Lung Cancer, https://en.wikipedia.org/wiki/Lung_cancer (Accessed 3/24/2017)

Witschi H (2001) A Short History of Lung Cancer. Toxicological Sciences 64: 4-6.

Chapter 6: Herbal Supplements and "Nutraceuticals"

Bailey RL, Gahche JJ, Lentino CV, Dwyer JT, Engel JS, Thomas PR, Betz JM, Sempos CT, Picciano MF (2011) Dietary supplement use in the United States, 2003-2006. Journal of Nutrition 141(2): 261-266.

Ballentine C (1981) Sulfanilamide Disaster. FDA Consumer Magazine, June 1981. (https://www.fda.gov/about-fda/histories-product-regulation/sulfanil-amide-disaster) (Accessed 6/5/2019)

FDA (2017) FDA warns consumers not to use Balguti Kesaria Ayurvedic Medicine due to high levels of lead. (https://www.fda.gov/drugs/drug-safety-and-availability/fda-warns-con-sumers-not-use-balguti-kesaria-ayurvedic-medicine-due-high-levels-lead) (Accessed 6/5/2019)

Krishna YR, Mittal V, Grewal P, Fiel MI, Schiano T. (2011) Acute liver failure caused by "fat burners" and dietary supplements: A case report and literature review. Canadian Journal of Gastroenterology 25(3): 157-160.

Long J (2017) FDA warns marketers of supplements and other products—Stop making cancer claims. Natural Products Insider, April 26, 2017 (https://www.naturalproductsinsider.com/blogs/insider-law/2017/04/fda-warns-mar-keters-of-supplements-and-other-prod.aspx) (Accessed 6/5/2019).

National Research Council (2005) Dietary Supplements: A Framework for Evaluating Safety. Committee on the Framework for Evaluating the Safety of Dietary Supplements, Food and Nutrition Board, Board on Life Sciences, Institute of Medicine, National Research Council, The National Academies Press, Washington, D.C. (www.nap.edu ; https://www.nap.edu/catalog/10882/dietary-supplements-a-framework-for-evaluating-safety) (Accessed 6/5/2019)

Navarro VJ, Bernhart H, Bonkovsky HL, Davern T, Fontana RJ, Grant L, Reddy KR, Seeff LB, Serrano J, Sherker AH, Stolz A, Talwalkar J, Vega M, Vuppalanchi R (2014) Liver injury from herbals and dietary supplements in the US Drug Induced Liver Injury Network. Hepatology 60(4): 1399-1408.

New York Times (2013) Spike in Harm to Liver Is Tied to Dietary Aids, December 22, Page A1.

Sugimura T (1982) Mutagens, carcinogens, and tumor promotors in our daily food. Cancer 49: 1970-1984.

Willett WC (1995) Diet, nutrition, and cancer. Environmental Health Perspectives 103 (Suppl. 8): 165-170.

U.S. Food and Drug Administration (2018) Dietary Supplements Guidance Documents & Regulatory Information, https://www.fda.gov/food/ guidance-documents-regulatory-information-topic-food-and-dietary-supplements/dietary-supplements-guidance-documents-regulatory-information#qhc (accessed 6/5/2019)

U.S. Food and Drug Administration (2019) New Dietary Ingredients (NDI) Notification Process, https://www.fda.gov/food/dietary-supplements/new-dietary-ingredients-ndi-notification-process (accessed 6/5/2019)

Chapter 7: Drug and Chemical Spiking of Nutraceuticals

Brackett RE (2006) Testimony before the Senate Committee on Government Reform, March 9, 2006 (https://www.fda.gov/NewsEvents/Testimony/ ucml12576.htm) (Accessed April 26, 2017, from FDA archives)

Cohen PA, Maller G, DeSouza, Neal-Kababick, J (2014) Presence of banned drugs in dietary supplements following FDA recalls. J. American Medical Association 312(16) 1691-1693. Doi: 10.1001/jama.2014.10308

FDA (2017) Vitamin Shop Owner Guilty of Selling Misbranded Drugs and Controlled Substance, Office of Criminal Investigations, U.S. Food and Drug Administration, May 15, 2017 (https://www.fda.gov/ICECI/ CriminalInvestigations/ucm558902.htm) (Accessed 5/30/2017)

Foster S (2011) A brief history of adulteration of herbs, spices, and botanical drugs. HerbalGram 92: 42-57. (http://cms.herbalgram.org/herbalgram/ issue92/FEAT-HxAdulteration.html)

Harnly JM, Luthria D, Chen P (2012) Detection of Adulterated *Ginkgo biloba* Supplements Using Chromatographic and Spectral Fingerprints. Journal of the AOAC 95(6): 1579–1587.

Schmidt E, Wanner J (2016) Adulteration of Essential Oils, in Handbook of Essential Oils, 2nd Edition, Ed. Hüsnü Can Başer K and Bachbauer G, CRC press, Boca Raton, FL, pp. 709-745.

Schultz H (2017) CVS to institute new testing requirements for dietary supplements. NutraIngredients-USA.com Newsletter, April 24, 2017 (http://www.nutraingredients-usa.com/Markets/CVS-to-institute-new-testing-requirements-for-dietary-supplements)

U.S. Food and Drug Administration (2018) How to Report a Problem with Dietary Supplements. https://www.fda.gov/food/ dietary-supplements/how-report-problem-dietary-supplements (Accessed 6/5/2019)

Wall Street Journal (2015) Oregon sues GNC, alleging supplements contained illegal ingredients, Oct. 22, 2015 (www.wsj.com/articles/oregon-sues-gnc-alleging-supplements-contained-illegal-ingredients-1445543143) (Accessed 4/26/2018)

Chapter 8: Regulation of Food Products, Additives, and Pesticide Residues

American Medical Association (2012) Bioengineered (Genetically Engineered) Crops and Foods H-480.958 (https://policysearch.ama-assn.org/policyfinder/detail/bioengineered%20foods?uri=%2FAMADoc%2FHOD.xml-0-4359.xml) (Accessed 6/6/2019)

Breuning G, Lyons JM (2000) The case of the FLAVR SAVR tomato. California Agriculture 54: 6-7. (http://calag.ucanr.edu/Archive/ ?article=ca.v054n04p6) (Accessed 6/6/2019)

Code of Federal Regulations, 21 CFR Chapter I, Subchapter B – FOOD FOR HUMAN CONSUMPTION, https://www.law.cornell.edu/cfr/text/21/chapter-I/subchapter-B (Accessed 6/6/2019)

Ellstrand NC (2003) Going to "great lengths" to prevent escape of genes that produce specialty chemicals. Plant Physiology 132(4): 1770-1774. (https://www.ncbi.nlm.nih.gov/pmc/articles/PMC526271/pdf/1321770.pdf) (Accessed 6/6/2019)

Funk C , Raine L (2015) Public and scientists' views on science and society. Pew Research center. January 2015 (www.pewinternet.org/2015/01/29/public-and-scientists-views-on-science-and-society) (Accessed 6/6/2019)

Kyndt T, Quispe D, Zhai H, Jarret R, Ghislain M, Liu Q, Gheysen G, Kreuze JF (2015) The genome of cultivated sweet potato contains *Agrobacterium* T-DNAs with expressed genes: An example of a naturally transgenic food crop. Proc. Nat. Acad. Sci. 112(18): 5844-5849.

Law Library of Congress (2014) Restrictions on Genetically Modified Organisms: United States. By Luis Acosta, www.loc.gov/law/help/restrictions-on-gmos/usa.php (Accessed 6/6/2019)

Naples Daily News (2017) Syngenta GMO Lawsuits to Begin, Section B, April 24, 2017.

National Corn Growers Association (2015) Viptera Corn Lawsuits, May 2015 (https://www.ncga.com/viptera-lawsuit-faq) (Accessed 6/6/2019)

National Archives (2019) Code of Federal Regulations, Title 21 List of Subjects, https://www.archives.gov/federal-register/cfr/subject-title-21.html (Accessed 6/6/2019)

OECD Guidelines: www.oecd-ilibrary.org; then search *"testing guidelines"*; then select *"health effects"*

OECD (2011) Consensus document on compositional considerations for new varieties of low erucic acid rapeseed (canola): key food and feed nutrients, anti-nutrients and toxicants Series on the Safety of Novel Foods and Feeds No. 24 JT03313855, OECD Environment Directorate Joint Meeting of the Chemicals Committee and the Working Party on Chemicals, Pesticides and Biotechnology, 23-Dec-2011. (https://www.oecd.org/env/ehs/bio-track/49343153.pdf) (Accessed 6/6/2019)

Society of Toxicology (2017) SOT Issue Statement of Food and Feed Safety of Genetically engineered Food Crops, (https://www.toxicology.org/pubs/statements/SOT_Safety_of_GE_Food_Crops_Issue_Statement_FINAL.pdf) (Accessed 6/6/2019)

U.S. Code of Federal Regulations. Title 21, Food and Drugs; Title 40, Protection of Environment; Title 7, Agriculture: (https://www.gpo.gov/fdsys/browse/collectionCfr.action?collection-Code=CFR) (Accessed 6/6/2019)

U.S. Code of Federal Regulations Subchapter M, Part 205, Organic Foods Production Act Provisions, Title 7, Subtitle B, Chapter I, Subchapter M (as defined in The Organic Foods Production Act of 1990, as amended (7 U.S.C. 6501 *et seq.*)), (2019) http://www.ecfr.gov/cgi-bin/text-idx?c=ecfr&sid=3f34f-4c22f9aa8e6d9864cc2683cea02&tpl=/ecfrbrowse/Title07/7cfr205_main_02.tpl (Accessed 6/6/2019)

USDA National Organic Program: http://www.ecfr.gov/cgi-bin/retrieveEC-FR?gp=&SID=1e4810996b1f6822e1653102bb278013&mc=true&n=pt7.3.205&r=PART&ty=HTML#se7.3.205_11 (Accessed 6/6/2019)

USDA Organic Regulations: https://www.ams.usda.gov/rules-regulations/organic (Accessed 6/6/2019)

U.S. Environmental Protection Agency (2017) Summary of the Federal Insecticide, Fungicide, and Rodenticide Act, https://www.epa.gov/ laws-regulations/summary-federal-insecticide-fungicide-and-rodenticide-act (Accessed 6/6/2019)

USDA (2017) National Organic Program – International Trade Arrangements and Agreements, Office of Inspector General, Audit Report 01601-0001-21, Washington, D.C. (https://www.usda.gov/oig/webdocs/01601-0001-21.pdf) (Accessed 6/6/2019)

U.S. Federal Food, Drug, and Cosmetic Act, https://www.fda.gov/regulatory-information/laws-enforced-fda/federal-food-drug-and-cosmetic-act-fdc-act (accessed 6/6/2019)

U.S. Food and Drug Administration (2007) Redbook 2000: Guidance for Industry and Other Stakeholders – Toxicological Principles for the Safety Assessment of Food Ingredients, Revised July 2007 (http://www.fda.gov/ Food/GuidanceRegulation/GuidanceDocumentsRegulatoryInformation/ IngredientsAdditivesGRASPackaging/ucm2006826.htm) (Accessed 6/6/2019)

U.S. Food and Drug Administration (2017) Draft Guidance for Industry: Regulation of Intentionally Altered Genomic DNA in Animals, Center for Veterinary Medicine, January 2017 (www.fda.gov/downloads/ AnimalVeterinary/GuidanceComplianceEnforcement/GuidanceforIndustry/ ucm113903.pdf) (Accessed 6/6/2019)

U.S. Food and Drug Administration (2018) How FDA regulates food from genetically engineered plants. https://www.fda.gov/food/food-new-plant-varieties/how-fda-regulates-food-genetically-engineered-plants (Accessed 6/6/2019)

U.S. Food and Drug Administration (2018) How to report a problem with dietary supplements (https://www.fda.gov/food/dietary-supplements/how-report-problem-dietary-supplements) (Accessed 6/6/2019)

U.S. Food and Drug Administration (2018) Federal Food, Drug, and Cosmetic Act (FD&C Act), FD&C Act Reference Information, United States Code, Title 21, https://www.fda.gov/regulatory-information/laws-enforced-fda/federal-food-drug-and-cosmetic-act-fdc-act (Accessed 6/6/2019)

U.S. Organic Foods Production Act of 1990, http://uscode.house.gov/view.xhtml?path=/prelim@title7/chapter94&edition=prelim (Accessed 6/6/2019)

Wikipedia (2018) Mutation breeding, https://en.wikipedia.org/wiki/Mutation_breeding, Edited Dec. 2018 (Accessed 6/6/2019)

Chapter 9: Regulation of Dietary Supplements, Pharmaceuticals, and Cosmetics

Ames BN, Profet M, Gold LS (1990) Nature's chemicals and synthetic chemicals: Comparative toxicology. Proceedings of the National Academy of Sciences, USA 87: 7782-7786. Available at: https://www.ncbi.nlm.nih.gov/pmc/articles/PMC54832/pdf/pnas01044-0445.pdf (Accessed 6/7/2019)

Dietary Supplement Health and Education Act of 1994, https://www.congress.gov/bill/103rd-congress/senate-bill/784/text (Accessed 6/7/2019)

Electronic Code of Federal Regulations (2019) Title 21, Chapter I, Subchapter C: Drugs; General (https://www.ecfr.gov/cgi-bin/text-idx?SID=1782402f92ddbcd92007ca8d566d98d5&mc=true&tpl=/ecfrbrowse/Title21/21CIsubchapC.tpl) (Accessed 6/7/2019)

FDA (2018) M7(R1) Assessment and Control of DNA Reactive (Mutagenic) Impurities in Pharmaceuticals to Limit Potential Carcinogenic Risk, Guidance for Industry, U.S. Department of Health and Human Services, Food and Drug Administration, Center for Drug Evaluation and Research (CDER), March 2018. Center for Drug Evaluation and Research, 10001 New Hampshire Ave., Hillandale Bldg., 4th Floor, Silver Spring, MD 20993. (https://www.fda.gov/ucm/groups/fdagov-public/@fdagov-drugs-gen/documents/document/ucm347725.pdf) (Accessed 6/7/2019)

Long J (2017) FDA supplement director seeking collaboration in developing pre-DSHEA list. Natural Products Insider, March 13, 2017. (www.

naturalproductsinsider.com/blogs/insider-law/2017/03/fda-supplement-director-seeking-collaboration-in.aspx) (Accessed March 23, 2017)

OECD Guidelines for safety testing of chemicals: www.oecd-ilibrary.org; then search *"testing guidelines"*; then select *"health effects"*

The International Conferences for Harmonisation of Technical Requirements for Pharmaceuticals for Human Use (ICH): www.ich.org; then select *"guidelines"* (Accessed 6/7/2019)

U.S. Federal Food, Drug, and Cosmetic Act, https://www.fda.gov/regulatory-information/laws-enforced-fda/federal-food-drug-and-cosmetic-act-fdc-act (accessed 6/7/2019)

U.S. Food and Drug Administration, Dietary Supplements (https://www.fda.gov/food/dietarysupplements/default.htm) (Accessed 6/7/2019)

U.S. Food and Drug Administration (2016) Draft Guidance for Industry: New Dietary Ingredient Notifications and Related Issues (https://www.fda.gov/regulatory-information/search-fda-guidance-documents/draft-guidance-industry-new-dietary-ingredient-notifications-and-related-issues   ) (Accessed 6/7/2019)

U.S. Food and Drug Administration (2018) Development & Approval Process (Drugs),   https://www.fda.gov/drugs/development-approval-process-drugs (Accessed 6/7/2019)

U.S. Food and Drug Administration (2018) FDA Authority Over Cosmetics: How cosmetics are not FDA-approved, but are FDA-regulated (https://www.fda.gov/cosmetics/cosmetics-laws-regulations/fda-authority-over-cosmetics-how-cosmetics-are-not-fda-approved-are-fda-regulated) (Accessed 6/7/2019)

Chapter 10: Burden of Proof

Bunge J and McKay B (2017) Anti-Zika insecticides approach "dead end". The Wall Street Journal, Friday, January 6.

Dallas News (2013) The risky business of dietary supplements. Dallas Morning News, Nov. 29, 2013 (www.dallasnews.com/opinion/sunday-commentary/20131129-the-risky-business-of-dietary-supplements.ece) (accessed 6/7/2019)

Schultz H (2017) Study finds "next DMAA" in tainted sports weight loss products. NutraIngredients-USA, November 9, 2017 (https://www.nutraingredients-usa.com/Article/2017/11/09/Study-finds-next-DMAA-in-tainted-sports-weight-loss-products) (Accessed 6/7/2019)

U.S. Food and Drug Administration (2013) DMAA in dietary supplements. U.S. Food and Drug Administration, Protecting and promoting your health, http://www.fda.gov/Food/DietarySupplements/ProductsIngredients/ucm346576.htm (Accessed 6/7/2019)

U.S. Food and Drug Administration (2014) Fiscal Year 2015 Justification of Estimates for Appropriations Committees, http://www.fda.gov/downloads/AboutFDA/ReportsManualsForms/Reports/BudgetReports/UCM388309.pdf (Accessed 12/18/2015)

U.S. Food and Drug Administration (2019) Fiscal Year 2020 Food and Drug Administration Justification of Estimates for Appropriations Committees, https://www.fda.gov/media/121408/ download (Accessed 6/10/2019)

Welsh S (2013) FDA: Dietary supplement dangerous, www.cnn.com/2013/04/15/health/fda-warning/ (Accessed 6/7/2019)

Chapter 12: What Really Matters

Blot WJ, Tarone RE (2015) Doll and Peto's quantitative estimates of cancer risks: Holding generally true for 35 years. J. National Cancer Institute 107(4): djv044 (doi: 10.1093/jnci/djv044) (https://academic.oup.com/jnci/article/107/4/djv044/894954) (Accessed June 11, 2019)

Centers for Disease Control and Prevention (2018) National Center for Chronic Disease Prevention and Health Promotion, Chronic Disease Data, https://www.cdc.gov/chronicdisease/data/index.htm (Accessed 6/11/2019)

Doll R, Peto R (1981) The causes of cancer: quantitative estimates of avoidable risks of cancer in the United States today. J. National Cancer Institute 66(6): 1191-1308.

Health Canada (2018) Canada's Food Guide Consultation – Phase 2 What We Heard Report. Summary of the Health Canada findings of the second open consultation for Canada's Food Guide, reflecting evidence related to healthy eating recommendations. (https://www.canada.ca/en/services/health/publications/food-nutrition/canada-food-guide-phase2-what-we-heard.html) (Accessed June 11, 2019)

Health Canada (2016) Evidence Review for Dietary Guidance: Summary of Results and Implications for Canada's Food Guide (https://www.canada.ca/en/health-canada/services/publications/food-nutrition/evidence-review-dietary-guidance-summary-results-implications-canada-food-guide.html) (Accessed June 11, 2019)

Physical Activity Guidelines Advisory Committee (2018) 2018 Physical Activity Guidelines Advisory Committee Scientific Report. Washington, DC: U.S. Department of Health and Human Services. (https://health.gov/paguidelines/second-edition/report/) (Accessed June 11, 2019)

Smith JC, Nielson KA, Antuono P, Lyons J-A, Hanson RJ, Butts AM, Hantke NC, Verber MD (2013) Semantic memory fMRI and cognitive function after exercise intervention in mild cognitive impairment. *Journal of Alzheimer's Disease*. 37(1) 197-215.

U.S. Department of Health and Human Services and U.S. Department of Agriculture. 2015–2020 Dietary Guidelines for Americans. 8th Edition. December 2015. Available at http://health.gov/dietaryguidelines/2015/guidelines/ (Accessed June 11, 2019)

U.S. Department of Health and Human Services. *2008 Physical Activity Guidelines for Americans*. Washington (DC): U.S. Department of Health and Human Services; 2008. ODPHP Publication No. U0036. Available at: http://www.health.gov/paguidelines. (Accessed June 11, 2019)

University of Maryland (2013) Exercise may be the best medicine for Alzheimer's disease. ScienceDaily, 30 July 2013. (www.sciencedaily.com/releases/2013/07/130730123249.htm) (Accessed June 11, 2019)

U.S. Food and Drug Administration, 2018 FDA Nutrition Innovation Strategy. (https://www.fda.gov/Food/LabelingNutrition/ucm602651.htm) (Accessed June 11, 2019)

U.S. Food and Drug Administration (2018) New and improved Nutrition Facts label, (https://www.fda.gov/food/nutrition-education-resources-and-materials/new-and-improved-nutrition-facts-label) (Accessed June 11, 2019)

U.S. Food and Drug Administration, Changes to the nutrition facts label. (https://www.fda.gov/food/food-labeling-nutrition/changes-nutrition-facts-label) (Accessed June 11, 2019)

Wikipedia. Sleep Deprivation. (https://en.wikipedia.org/wiki/Sleep_deprivation) (Accessed June 11, 2019)

Wikipedia, Effects of sleep deprivation on cognitive performance.(https://en.wikipedia.org/wiki/Effects_of_sleep_deprivation_on_cognitive_performance) (Accessed June 11, 2019)

Willett WC (1995) Diet, nutrition, and avoidable cancer. Environmental Health Perspectives 103(Suppl. 8): 165-170.